Go Green Get Lean

Trim Your Waistline with the Ultimate Low-Carbon Footprint Diet

KATE GEAGAN, MS, RD

RODALE

This book is intended as a reference volume only, not as a medical manual. The information given here is designed to help you make informed decisions about your health. It is not intended as a substitute for any treatment that may have been prescribed by your doctor. If you suspect that you have a medical problem, we urge you to seek competent medical help.

The information in this book is meant to supplement, not replace, proper exercise training. All forms of exercise pose some inherent risks. The editors and publisher advise readers to take full responsibility for their safety and know their limits. Before practicing the exercises in this book, be sure that your equipment is well-maintained, and do not take risks beyond your level of experience, aptitude, training, and fitness. The exercise and dietary programs in this book are not intended as a substitute for any exercise routine or dietary regimen that may have been prescribed by your doctor. As with all exercise and dietary programs, you should get your doctor's approval before beginning. Mention of specific companies, organizations, or authorities in this book does not imply endorsement by the author or publisher, nor does mention of specific companies, organizations, or authorities imply that they endorse this book, its author, or the publisher.

Internet addresses and telephone numbers given in this book were accurate at the time it went to press.

Rodale books may be purchased for business or promotional use or for special sales. For information, please write to:

Special Markets Department, Rodale Inc., 733 Third Avenue, New York, NY 10017

Printed in the United States of America
Rodale Inc. makes every effort to use acid-free ∞, recycled paper ♻.

Interior design by Carol Angstadt
Cover design by Christopher Rhoads

Library of Congress Cataloging-in-Publication Data

Geagan, Kate.
    Go green, get lean : trim your waistline with the ultimate low-carbon footprint diet / Kate Geagan.
      p.   cm.
    Includes bibliographical references.
    ISBN-13 978–1–60529–989–1 pbk.
    ISBN-10 1–60529–989–8 pbk.
    1. Reducing diets—Environmental aspects. 2. Natural foods. 3. Organic living. I. Title.
    RM222.2.G424 2009
    613.2'5—dc22   2008047320

Distributed to the trade by Macmillan

2 4 6 8 10 9 7 5 3 1   paperback

RODALE
LIVE YOUR WHOLE LIFE™

We inspire and enable people to improve their lives and the world around them
For more of our products visit **rodalestore.com** or call 800-848-4735

FOR GEORGIA AND CHASE,
THE ABSOLUTE BEST
NOURISHMENT OF ALL

CONTENTS

PART V. WHITTLE YOUR WAISTLINE WITH SUSTAINABLE SIPPING

PART VI. TREADING MORE LIGHTLY—FOREVER

ACKNOWLEDGMENTS

This book would have truly been impossible without the unwavering support of clients, friends, colleagues, and my management team. Julie May, my manager, you are the best; thank you for your vision, your encouragement, and your ability to turn my dreams into reality. I am honored to call you not only my manager but a friend as well.

To Mary Lengle, my publicist, whose steadfast belief in this project and in me has empowered me to take new risks. To Shea Zukowski, editor extraordinaire, whose energy and enthusiasm from our very first meeting for this book made it crystal clear that you were the perfect person to help me bring this project to the world. Thank you for your dedication, your ability to keep me closely on track with our vision, and your commitment to creating the best book possible. I am eternally grateful. And to Julie Will, who helped me make it to the finish line, thank you.

To all of my clients, colleagues, and friends who have contributed quotations, feedback, and encouragement for this project at every step of the way. I am grateful for all your support in helping to bring this book to fruition. This book is for you.

For my professional colleagues Felicia Stoler, Lisa Stevenson, Mitzi Dulan, Christopher Speed, Amanda Archibald, Dina Aronson, Katherine Kwon, Gail Funstra, and Vicki Shanta-Retelny, who took time to provide valuable feedback and professional insights, as well as to sharpen ideas and provide much-needed encouragement at many steps of the process. I simply couldn't have done it without you; thank you for your support and guidance, all of you. To my amazing intern Ryann Collins; your help in combing through the details was the best, and I am indebted to you.

To Melanie Plesko, Keith Snow, and Jennifer Watson, exceptional chefs who generously lent time and professional expertise and shared their recipes with me without hesitation. I am grateful for your help in providing concrete expert cooking suggestions to make leaner and greener living within the grasp of everyone.

To my family: Pete, for being my rock, for believing in me from the very start, and for helping to create the space in our lives for "the year of the book." Without you, this literally would not have been possible. To Bob Hopper and Sarah Johnson, for helping me push beyond "this is a great book idea" into action. It is because of your encouragement and insights that this book ever got moving from dream into reality. And to my sister Eileen, for the hours you pored over my notes and drafts, providing feedback and sharing "real life" questions; I am so grateful for your belief in me, and for the time you devoted to help me make this book the best it could be. To Lalo, for your help in dressing me for success when I went to New York to pitch this idea to publishers, and to Jeff for "getting it" right away and being so supportive from the very start. And to my mom and dad, David and Jade Walsh, you have always encouraged me to follow my passions, telling me that the best way to find professional success was to do something I loved. I love you for giving me what is perhaps that greatest gift of all; this book is because of you. And most important, for Georgia and Chase, the inspirations for and driving force behind this entire project; you two are by far my life's best nourishment.

INTRODUCTION

"Knowing where your food comes from can change your life."

—Alice Waters

I wrote this book for my children.

As a dietitian with a successful corporate wellness practice, I had worked with thousands of people to help them lose weight, manage chronic disease, and improve their health through diet. I loved staying abreast of the latest clinical research on food findings, and then helping my clients incorporate the newest proven strategies or foods for effectively managing weight, fighting disease, and feeding their families soundly, while helping companies better manage their spiraling health-care costs.

Then I had children, and my world changed. Suddenly the issue of global health, always important but somehow easy to nudge into the backseat of day-to-day life, took on a clearer focus. In fact, there was an exact moment when I knew I was going to write this book. I refer to it as "my PB&J moment."

It was the summer of 2007, and I was at the playground with my kids and several other moms and tots. After about an hour, we all pulled out snacks. I watched with fascination as one mom pulled out a premade, frozen, prepackaged, crustless PB&J on white bread, cut neatly into a little white circle and prewrapped in a clear plastic package. It was a little diskette of technology, convenience, and "food product" for a little boy to snack on.

In truth, this particular mom, like all of us, was only trying to do the best thing for her kids while balancing a time-strapped reality. And up until that moment, I had been equally guilty in other ways, such as breezily making suggestions to clients to load up on single-serving, pre-portioned (which meant calorie-controlled) items as a dieter's manna from Skinny Heaven.

But here's a rundown of what went through my head at that moment:

- Have we really gotten to the point where making a 30-second PB&J seems too time-consuming? Worth outsourcing to someone else?

- How much fossil fuel was that snack drenched in, from the automated production at the plant, to the packaging of each of the sandwiches, to the cardboard box with splashy marketing, to plunging the box into a deep freeze, to shipping the frozen product (they are in the freezer aisle) to the supermarket, to sitting in the freezer aisle at the supermarket until this mom drove to pick it up, then stored it in her freezer until she decided that her kid might want a snack in an hour and she popped it into her diaper bag to thaw out so he could have it?

- How many thousands of other snacks and foods like this are lining supermarket shelves around the country?

- If she's truly trying to do what's best for her child, is this really what she has been led to believe? Might she make a different choice if she saw things from another perspective?

This "PB&J moment" got me thinking deeply over the next couple of days about the connection between the grocery aisle and Antarctica's glaciers. Could it be a lot closer than we realize? I decided to investigate further to see if I could make some different suggestions to clients to help them eat in a greener way.

And what I found appalled me.

The American diet is warming the planet.

Americans' food choices are a significant driver of the global warming crisis.

Yes, it is our *food choices,* and all of the energy that it takes to give us these choices (including production, transport, processing, packaging, storage, and preparation), that is now the single largest contributor to global warming, eclipsing even our love affair with our SUVs. The average American diet creates 2.8 tons of CO_2 emissions each year per person, *which has now surpassed the 2.2 tons generated by Americans driving.*[1]

The impact of these choices is now echoing around the globe, not just because our food is nowadays logging more frequent-flier miles than we are, with blueberries from Argentina and grapes from Chile, but because throughout the whole system of food production, from when it is produced to when we put it in our mouths, the amount of fossil fuel going into our food choices has outstripped the actual amount of energy in the food itself. Even something as seemingly innocuous as lettuce can require a river of petroleum to bring it to diners' plates; the average head of lettuce grown in California and picked at the peak of ripeness ends up requiring nearly 60 calories of fossil fuel for every food calorie by the time it arrives on a diner's plate in New York City.[2] This is to say nothing of the thousands of highly processed foods that require barrels of oil to create but provide little return in terms of real nutrition.

So thus begins a new chapter in the diet debate. Your food choices not only determine the current (and future) state of your health and weight but are also a significant portion of your overall carbon footprint that will affect future generations. And the typical American diet has the global impact of a Hummer. Further, that same diet is clogging their arteries, fattening their waistlines, and wreaking havoc on their immune systems.

The good news is that you can enjoy health, flavor, and a genuine excitement for food while cutting your carbon footprint. You do not have to subsist on reconstituted gruel and local twigs in order to trim the amount of fossil fuel on your plate. In fact, I was inspired to create this eating plan precisely because it is easy, is doable, and can have significant health and carbon impacts *now*; you will lose weight and lighten your carbon load at the same time. Believe me, as someone living high in the Wasatch Mountains in Utah, if anyone was scared about the "pleasure" implications of cutting a carbon footprint (did I mention I am a foodie obsessed with authentic ingredients such as prosciutto di Parma *from* Parma, Italy?), it was me.

So here's how it works.

You will enjoy a variety of fruits, vegetables, lean proteins, and grains.

You will eat at a better spot on the food chain, one that cuts your waist *and* your waste (and you'll still get to enjoy that steak once in a while).

You'll live a bit more like a locavore (eating more local and seasonal food) when your area's growing season allows it.

You'll realign your relationship with industrial food.

You will move your kids from "food products" back to real food in a way that's easy, tasty, and still fun.

You'll still get to savor dessert and alcohol in moderation.

While doing all this, you will *also* significantly cut your carbon impact. In fact, what makes this book unique is that you can use it not only as a diet book, but also as a guide to actively green up your diet and cut greenhouse gases associated with your food choices.

So that is the genesis for this book. And I hope you will join me. While the global warming crisis is admittedly complicated, with many far-reaching tentacles that need to be sorted out, *one of the largest, most significant tentacles (our food system) has a clear, easy, and immediate solution*. And the best part is that adapting the diet plan in this book can help you slim down, lean up, and dramatically reduce your odds of many chronic diseases, including the leading killers of heart disease and diabetes. If you have children, it will help them change course from being what the Centers for Disease Control and Prevention (CDC) has warned could be "the first generation not to outlive their parents" to healthy, nourished eaters who enjoy real food instead of the "food product" that seems to have overtaken their lunch boxes and their lives.

Only *action* creates *results*. I implore you to join me in this "lean and green" revolution that will help you lose weight, cut your risk of disease, and significantly cut your carbon footprint *now*.

I think our children would be proud of us.

PART I

THE NEW
LEAN AND GREEN
CUISINE

CHAPTER 1

AN INCONVENIENT TOOTH

Our Food Choices Are Making Us Fat and Hastening Climate Change

"You eat. Willingly or not, you participate in the environment of food choice. The choices you make about food are as much about the kind of world you want to live in as they are about what to have for dinner. Food choices are about your future and that of your children."

—Marion Nestle, *What to Eat*

The American diet is in an energy crisis.

Whether we're talking about food calories or energy use, our penchant for overconsumption is what has defined us both here and abroad as the American Consumer. More than two out of three Americans are overweight; one in three Americans is obese; and we use 25 percent of the world's oil though we represent only 5 percent of the world's population.

Like a giant snowball, Americans have tried to push the consequences of our choices as far off into the distance as we could, be they poor eating habits, an energy-intense lifestyle, or even poor money management. Unfortunately, those snowballs are beginning to collapse under their own weight and come to a creaking halt.

Experts tell us that Americans' food choices reflect what is easy, cheap, and tasty, and brings us immediate pleasure. Such a dietary lifestyle is one of the reasons our health-care system is saddled with chronic disease; heart disease, diabetes, hypertension, and obesity have become so commonplace and are thus such an integral part of our health-care costs and drug regimens that it's easy to forget that these diseases are largely preventable. In many parts of the world that practice different eating habits, their incidence is dramatically lower. These diseases are, for the most part, a direct result of the daily food and lifestyle choices we make as the American Consumer. These are diseases of affluence.

On the other side of the coin lies the paradox—namely, that the heaviest nation on the planet is also the most weight obsessed. We seek easy, fast, painless solutions to our weight woes, with Americans spending the most money per capita on losing weight; in 2005 alone, we shelled out more than $35 billion in search of quick fixes. Each year we flock in record numbers to weight-loss centers and the supplement aisle in search of a cure. Yet despite these efforts, our bathroom scales continue to creep steadily upward.

In contrast to the rest of the world, where local food pathways and national cuisines have grown out of deep cultural underpinnings, the United States is unique in that its food landscape has been shaped in large part by marketers and food companies. Much of this cultural shift began after World War II, on the heels of advances made in food processing, packaging, and distribution during the war, and with the explosion of Madison Avenue to direct our food choices and our relationship to the kitchen. The message was clear: Hurry out of the kitchen, and let Betty Crocker (or some other equally friendly persona) do the cooking for you. Processed food was the future. What could be more convenient?

As a result, the typical Western eating pattern that has emerged is heavy in red meat and processed meats, refined grains and sugars, and animal fats such as butter, cheese, and ice cream; it relies on processed food products and convenience foods; and it's overflowing with high-calorie sweetened beverages that are basically liquid candy. It is also low in whole grains, beans, fruits and vegetables, and fish. This diet not only makes us fat but also leads us directly to numerous chronic diseases; it saps our energy and vitality, but it also turns out to be a Hummer of an eating style.

Therein lies the double energy crisis of our current food situation—far too many food calories brought to us in foods that are extremely energy intense to make. Americans, it is becoming clear, have an inconvenient tooth. A big one.

Our SUV-style diet is warming the planet. All of the steps it takes to bring that fast-food burger, that low-carb frozen dinner, even that organic asparagus from Argentina to your plate require fossil fuel. And while we've begun to realize the physical consequences of our diet choices, the *global warming consequences* of our choices are no less serious. Over the past 20 years, we have been steadily marching toward an American diet that is more drenched in fossil fuel than any key nutrient.

On a global scale, food transportation is now among the biggest and fastest-growing sources of greenhouse gas emissions. Overall, more than 800 million tons of food are shipped around the planet each year, four times as many as in the 1960s. Just stop and think about the considerable miles our food travels, much of the time in either a cozily refrigerated or frozen truck bay. Here in the United States, food is traveling 25 percent farther than it did just 20 years ago (the average trip hovers somewhere between 1,500 and 2,500 miles from farm to table). The 2005 EPA report on US greenhouse gas emissions noted that the combustion of fossil fuels (which makes up 94 percent of national CO_2 emissions) has climbed more than 20 percent since 1990. One of the fundamental factors driving this is our globalized supermarket.

Need more data? Consider the following. Experts estimate that with our current food habits, it now takes roughly 7 to 10 calories of fossil fuel energy to bring 1 calorie of food energy to the American plate. That translates into 14,000 to 20,000 calories of fossil fuel per person per day if we're talking about the 2,000-calorie "standard intake" printed on nutrition facts labels everywhere—even more if you consider all that's wasted.

Most of my clients are shocked when I tell them our food system consumes nearly 20 percent of all petroleum that's burned annually in the United States. Sure, we may be thinking about energy-efficient fleets or energy-efficient buildings, but energy-efficient pantries? That's a new idea for most people. Fortunately, greening your pantry is a surprisingly easy change to make, and it will reap as big if not bigger savings to your personal carbon footprint as many of the other changes being put forward.

In fact, in terms of impact, your dietary lifestyle sits right up there with the type of car you drive. A 2005 study from the University of Chicago found that the greenhouse gas burden of a typical red meat diet compared to the diet of a plant eater equals the difference between driving a Camry and an SUV. If you're not ready to become a vegan, that's certainly okay (you're not alone), but you can still significantly cut back on our national warming trend by realigning your diet a bit. This same study found that simply ratcheting down the portion of animal-derived calories you eat each day can get you out of the SUV and into a more efficient sedan (while a vegan diet is the equivalent of an ultra-efficient hybrid). How fantastic, because this advice also overlaps exceedingly well with a clear and easy strategy for losing weight, reducing inflammation, and increasing your energy level, resulting in a fresh, lean and green cuisine that gives new meaning to the idea of "energy efficient."

Perhaps never before has the call been so strong, so clear, that we need a paradigm shift away from maximum efficiency and productivity toward sustainability. A shift away from extolling shelf life and convenience, because these "improvements" are actually undermining our quality of life. And to rediscover clean, simple nourishment in the form of clean, simple foods.

Now, if you're like most people, this carbon thing is something you probably haven't been considering while shopping the supermarket shelves, sampling the sundries in the vending machine at work, or sneaking into that fast-food burger joint on your way home. After all, our food system's role in the climate crisis hasn't been a central part of the discussion. Until now.

While the past decade has brought a rush of frankly written exposés, documentaries, and editorial pieces about our environment, as well as the deplorable state of our health and weight, we have been slow to see how the two crises intersect.

The question is, How much petroleum did your food require to get to your plate? The following chart outlines the steps that virtually all food goes through before landing on your plate; however, as the next several chapters will show, your choices can make an impact because the amount of fuel needed at each phase varies enormously; an apple from your local farmers' market (even a local apple that is sold in your local supermarket), for instance, requires far less oil on average than an apple shipped in a refrigerated cargo plane 3,000 miles from New Zealand.

How Much Fossil Fuel Did Your Lunch Require?

Our modern food system is built within the framework of an industrial economy. As a result, many foods drift through a river of petroleum before landing on your plate; consider the typical path in this chart and how fossil fuels are associated with each step in the process:

HEATING/COOLING

To ensure food safety and preservation during transport, most foods are brought to some ideal temperature/humidity immediately after harvesting. Just like heating and cooling a house, this step requires energy.

PRODUCTION

Fuel is required for many agricultural inputs (including growing feed and producing fertilizers and pesticides) as well as for cultivation and irrigation, labor, and equipment.

HARVEST

The vast majority of harvesting today is dependent on fossil fuel–powered equipment, whether in field, feedlot, ocean, farm, greenhouse, or slaughterhouse.

TRANSPORTATION

This facet of the process may also occur at multiple stages. For example, corn may be transported to a storage facility, then to a processing plant where it is made into corn syrup, which is then sent to another factory that uses the corn syrup as an ingredient in a frozen dessert that is shipped frozen to a freezer aisle near you. Or consider something like sushi, which may be caught fresh and airfreighted to the buyer so as to be as fresh as possible.

PROCESSING

Processing can occur at several points throughout the chain, and the amount of energy required varies widely (e.g., a fresh fish fillet requires very little processing, while a frozen fish dinner requires significantly more). Factors at play include labor and equipment, waste management, and packaging.

STORAGE

Few grocery stores receive all their products directly from manufacturers. Most have regional warehouses where products are processed for distribution. More equipment, heating, and cooling costs accumulate here.

FINAL DELIVERY AND PURCHASE

A New Paradigm:
Determining Your "Dietary Lifestyle"

When you start to calculate all the hidden costs involved in the food system, it's easy to see your "dietary lifestyle" emerge. And given our vast geography and access to tens of thousands of foods, your lifestyle might look more like either an SUV or a hybrid in terms of how much carbon your choices put into the atmosphere. Diets heavy in red meat, dairy products, processed foods, foods that require refrigeration to travel long distances, and imported ingredients are the Hummers of eating styles. So go ahead. Ask yourself, Does your diet resemble a Hummer or a hybrid?

Wherever your present diet leaves you on this continuum, here's the new reality: Your food choices are no longer just about you. This isn't about willpower or about fancy tricks to fool your biology into thinking you're full on cabbage soup. This is about an inconvenient tooth that America has collectively acquired, and how it's undermining our future, our health, and the planet. If you are looking for real answers to your weight problems, if you are passionate or concerned about global warming and want to be part of the solution rather than part of the problem, you need to start changing your eating habits. And collectively, we need to expand our thinking as to what is "healthy food" beyond simply the ingredient list or calorie count.

From what I have seen firsthand in my work as a corporate wellness dietitian, I think Americans are ready to change their food choices. Across the country I see people who are tired of being tired (oftentimes a direct result of poor eating habits), who are tired of worrying about their children's weight problems (oftentimes a direct result of poor eating habits), and most of all, who are tired of being overweight. Another benefit? Eating green is cheaper. In fact, the economic decline of 2008 has already moved some people back to a greener dietary lifestyle—you'll see precisely how in the upcoming chapters.

My mission is to help you look better, feel better, and eat better and, in doing so, to create a ripple effect that will help ensure we leave a better planet for our children. It's time to be frank about the state of our plate; the idea of "farm to plate," for most consumers today, is little more than a quaint notion or a reassuring sound bite. In reality, "package to palm," "microwave to couch," or "farm factory to drive-thru" would be a much more accurate description when it comes to Americans' relationship to food.

So what does the flip side of the coin look like? A lean and green eating pattern is a primarily plant-based diet rich in whole grains, seasonal and local fruits and vegetables, moderate amounts of chicken and fish or wild game, and very limited red meat. Organic foods are emphasized where it matters most, and sustainable splurges such as chocolate and wine are still deliciously included. This diet is lower in calories, packs far greater amounts of protective nutrients, is higher in fiber, and is much more energy efficient in every sense.

To get a stronger taste of just how vast our current global food system is, take a look at the map on page 10 from a project underway at Middlebury College in Vermont. It is a snapshot of just one meal served in their dining hall on one day. In one of the first projects of its kind, students used GIS (Geographic Information Systems) to track an entire supply chain from farm to college dining plate. Even the map of a college such as Middlebury that is at the forefront of sourcing locally (hey, they have all those great cows and dairies at their disposal) still looks like one of those confusing maps you find in the back of an in-flight magazine that shows all the different flight plans. The college's geography department is currently working on the next extension: How did the food get to the suppliers? What were those inputs? Where did the packaging come from? No doubt that version will be far more complicated.

"A food map is a stunning interactive representation of just how vast the global food system is," said Chris Howell, the Middlebury alum who developed the project after attending a "slow foods" event in Italy in 2006. "Food mapping helps people understand how our individual and institutional food choices play out environmentally, economically, socially, and politically. Imagine if your fast-food meal or shopping cart had such a map—what would it look like?"

So given all this new information, how do we respond? How do we continue to feed ourselves and our families in a way that is delicious, easy, and doable, without jeopardizing the ability of our children and grandchildren to do the same? Admittedly, it's not always easy to make decisions that are perfectly aligned with conscience; while you may be filled with good intentions to unleash your inner "eco-goddess," you may be waylaid by your child (or your own inner child) who is having a tantrum because she wants to go to McDonald's.

You respond by taking action anyway.

You respond by knowing that you won't be "perfect," but you can certainly be "much, much improved."

You respond by recognizing that you may need to rethink your definition of "splurge" when it comes to food. Need some more encouragement? Let's consider all there is to gain.

A Fresh Start:
The Health Benefits of Going Green

The best part about incorporating this fresh green cuisine into your diet is that every day you will serve up some of the best medicine

HOW FAR DID YOUR MEAL TRAVEL?

The Distance for *One* Meal at the Middlebury College Dining Hall

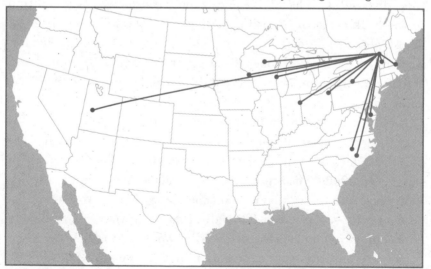

Courtesy of Professor Bill Hegman, geography department, Middlebury College. Reprinted with permission.

Mother Nature has to offer in the fight against fat, aging, inflammation, and chronic disease. It's a win-win. In fact, a 2008 study determined that by simply reducing the amount of meat and junk food in their diets, as well as supporting a return to more locally grown foods, Americans could see massive savings on the nation's fuel consumption and see big health benefits to boot.[1] And perhaps most surprisingly, you are likely to actually save more money as you adopt the strategies in this book, all without adding hours to the time you spend feeding yourself and your family. A recent study by UCLA, for example, found that "convenience" foods (which usually cost more per unit and are more heavily processed) aren't the time-savers you think they are when it comes to getting dinner on the table; they save only about 10 minutes of prep time over foods prepared the traditional way and shed zero time off total cooking.

The Go Green Get Lean Diet can be used on several different fronts. First, it is a powerful program for effective weight loss and for packing your diet with foods that have been shown to slow aging, reduce your risk of many of the leading diseases that plague Americans, and fight inflammation, even if you don't really care all that much about global warming (although I doubt you'd be reading this if that were the case).

It also stands on its own as a guide for a greener diet that lightens the fossil fuel load of your eating habits and reduces your carbon footprint. Perhaps you're not really interested in weight loss, but you are committed to eating in a more sustainable way. Or maybe you've greened up your house, your wheels, your energy sources, and your family vacations, and now you wonder, "What's next?" Here is what's next—your food!

If you're already following another eating plan with good success but want to green up your existing diet, you can also simply use the Lean and Green Prescriptions to see which choices from your allowed foods (on your current plan) are better bets for the planet, and then make the swap.

While the following chapters spell out each food group in detail and give you action steps, here are some "big picture" ways that going green also helps you go lean.

- A greener diet is based more heavily on plants (in general, plant production uses significantly less fossil fuel input than animal production does), which means more disease-fighting, antiaging nutrients in your diet (but rest assured, you do *not* have to become a vegetarian if you like eating meat).

- A greener diet is lower in total calories (ounce for ounce, plants have fewer calories than animal products), which trims excess weight.

- A greener diet contains fewer liquid calories, one of the biggest sources of "empty calories" and excess sugars in the American diet, which trims excess weight.

- A greener diet is *cost-effective* because it doesn't require you to purchase premade convenience foods, snack packs, bars, or shakes. It also realigns your shopping cart in a way that purges some of the highest-priced items per pound and replaces them with much cheaper yet healthier food choices.

- A greener diet is apt to be *safer* for you and your family because it involves fewer harmful pesticides and chemicals, hormones, and antibiotics. It also begins to wean you from an overreliance on a food production system vulnerable to large-scale contamination outbreaks.

- A greener diet is *easy to follow* because it gives you a simple, consistent framework for choice, eliminating the mind-boggling (and often conflicting) information consumers are barraged with on nearly every food label in today's supermarket.

Start Cleaner Living NOW

So when can you get started? Right now. Consider this to be your starting point.

In my years spent counseling people on how to lose weight, I've seen firsthand that for many people, there is often a lapse between *awareness* and *action*—in other words, people know what they should be doing, but they just don't *do* it, either because they are waiting for more information, trying to get their minds in the right place to commit, or have three excuses as to why they'll wait until Monday, until after the holidays, or until some other vaguely defined point in the future to begin making changes in their lives. But the state of the planet is now at a tipping point. The world is in crisis, and there are no excuses to sit on the sidelines anymore.

For that reason, I've designed this diet with a "Take Action Now" phase to get you *acting* right away, as well as to get you *losing* right away; that way, while you're still learning about a lean and green lifestyle, you are already on your way to changing your carbon footprint for the better and shedding some extra pounds.

While there are few quick fixes for the global warming dilemma, your diet offers a surprisingly large number of things you can do to have an immediate impact on your own personal rate of carbon burn, changes that will also start paying big dividends right away for your health and weight.

This book will help you decode the mind-boggling haze of food choices and "green" issues around your food, and provide specific metrics (where they exist) along the way, so you can know your impact.

Before we begin, let's get a few disclaimers out of the way.

- This book begins from the assumption that if you are reading it, you recognize the existence of the climate change crisis, you believe that our current choices and behaviors are warming the planet, and you are looking for something *you* can do *now* to have a significant impact on cutting your carbon footprint. It is not within the scope of this book to make the case that global warming is real, and that it is largely driven by human activities.

■ Literally as I type, the food landscape is changing. Some companies are changing their deepest paradigms to be part of the solution; others are swapping LEDs in the drive-thru sign and calling it green. This book will give you a road map to know how to snuff out dietary "greenwashing" and how to recognize real improvement in our food system and how you interact with it.

■ It is true that all food choices contribute some level of carbon footprint to Earth's atmosphere. Food is a basic need for all humans, and there will admittedly be impact just by nature of the fact that we need to grow food for everyone, and everyone doesn't live next to a farm. Therefore, as I see it, the issue rather becomes how we can significantly *cut* that footprint in a way that also trims our waistlines and minimizes our risk of disease, all while keeping food easy, delicious, and one of the fundamental pleasures of life. We need to invest in the future of great green cuisine now.

■ When I set out to write this book, I was hoping that there would be some wonderful database chronicling the petroleum journey of each piece of food produced, some super-cool "carbon footprint calculator" for every food choice under the sun, adjusted for whether I bought it fresh or frozen, whether it was already cooked at the store or whether I zapped it in my microwave at home, even whether I walked to buy my groceries or whether I drove in an SUV.

Unfortunately, while there are some organizations collecting important data to get us closer to that point, right now no such comprehensive database exists. Instead,

I have relied on the most recent figures from scientists and researchers who examine the impacts of the entire food supply chain. Thanks to groups such as the Carbon Disclosure Project and others, such databases may well exist in the future. In fact, many global food and retail companies are at this point simply trying to get their arms around their own total carbon footprint impact, leaving the consumer's role still in somewhat undefined terms. But if you are like most of the clients I have worked with over the years, you love seeing numbers—swap *this,* save *that,* eat *this,* and take an SUV off the road. I have done my best to provide you with those types of facts, so you can gauge both nutrition and carbon improvements.

One thing I have learned in my interviews and hundreds of hours of research: It is almost always possible to find a "yeah, but" in the dialogue about greener choices. Food is no exception. In a land that stretches from sea to shining sea, everyone's realities are different.

Here's another parallel: In the field of nutrition, the edges of the exact health debate seem to waver from time to time (Does fiber protect against colon cancer? Will selenium cut your risk of heart disease?), yet the basic building blocks of longer, more vital living have remained consistent (people who eat more fruits and vegetables are healthier than people who don't). It's the same with the carbon questions around your plate. Is that organic tomato from five states away a net carbon win over the conventional one you picked up at the farmers' market? The short answer: Don't get bogged down about being off a carbon point or two. Because while there is still much to be sorted out, there *are* some big, broad themes that we *do* know are critical when it comes to low-carbon eating. This book has been designed around those very themes (which, again, happen to overlap exceedingly well with a winning nutrition prescription). Stick to my lean and green guidelines and know that you're creating a powerful synergy that will get you shedding excess weight and carbon, even if some small exceptions can be found along the way.

■ You will see that many of the "greenest" recommendations for each food often include words such as "organic," "local," "grass fed," and "authentic." As a nutritionist and dietitian, my job is to point you in the direction of the very best foods for your very best health. And as you will soon see, these foods represent the best for a variety of reasons. However, if you can't find or afford all organic all the time (as I and many of my clients can't), don't sweat it. Focus on the areas where it's most important to your health (starting, in my opinion, with any animal products you consume) and just fill in the rest as you can. Week by week, I'll give you clear steps to help you scout out what is available in your area. No matter where you live (and I live in the high desert in Utah, so it doesn't get much harder than that), you will be amazed at some of the lean and green options that are closer to home than you realized. It's an exciting piece of this journey, and one that will pay big dividends in health, taste, and pleasure of food for years to come.

My view is simple. The philosophical core of what I am advocating flows from abundance, not deprivation. It flows from a deeper sense of stewardship for our bodies and our planet. We dietitians seem to get a bad rap as always wagging a finger, telling people what they can't have, and trying to get people ecstatic at the prospect of subsisting on things like carrot sticks and fat-free rice cakes forever. Think of me instead as an excited nutrition coach and friend, showing you what you should be eating more of, giving you the tools and resources you need to make these foods taste fresh and satisfying, and (like a good friend would) calling you out on the stuff you should be eating less of. Stuff that, if you're honest with yourself, you probably already know you should be eating less of anyway.

Of course, you are free to choose to eat however you wish; freedom of choice is an inalienable right and a defining value of the American dream. But when it comes to food, infinite choices and value pricing have a cost. My guess is, if you're truly honest with yourself, you could list some of the current costs you're already paying—such as reduced energy, a body you are dissatisfied with, or a chronic ailment that you manage with medication. In my counseling practice, I've seen firsthand the burdens of this limitless choice on individuals, but I have also seen the surprising shift that happens when people start to shed the burdens of excessive choice. In this age of excess and access, people are actually discovering a sense of liberation and finding their lives ultimately improved when they have a meaningful framework from which to operate, particularly in the realm of food. In the end, it's pretty simple. Don't believe what the food companies tell you—an abundance of choice is not *always* a better thing.

Now let's get started losing.

CHAPTER 2

WHAT'S TO GAIN BY LOSING

66 The Go Green Get Lean Diet helped me lose 12 pounds in about 2 months, and it's stayed off. It's just part of my lifestyle now. Kate has figured out all the nutritional complexities, leaving her clients with a simple road map to shed extra pounds and get healthy. This book is fascinating. With Kate's help, I'm leaner and greener. And I love that red wine is part of the secret. . . . 99

—Nick Seifert, outdoor television personality,
president, Fischer Productions, LLC

So what's to gain by losing?

Or, to put it a tad less eloquently, like the blogger named "Sugar-Daddy," who recently posted: "Hah. You can't even get people to save their own fat arses. I highly doubt that if you tell them it's for the good of the environment that it will be any different."

SugarDaddy's post (not to me personally, but to a 2008 report in *Human Ecology*) got me thinking. Why *do* I think this knowledge will trigger change in people, if data shows that currently only a small percentage of Americans are actively changing their habits in response to global warming? The answers came to me on many different levels.

First of all, because unlike squeezing onto a steamy, crowded bus in the name of saving the planet, there's an immediate personal benefit to gain by greener eating—namely, weight loss and improved energy. *And the reality is that people are more likely to change if they see an immediate benefit to themselves.*

Further, this easy solution also connects to another issue close to home that most Americans care deeply about: our kids. The Centers for Disease Control and Prevention (CDC) predicts that one out of three children born in 2000 or later will be saddled with type 2 diabetes as a direct result of our unhealthy food and lifestyle choices. The Go Green Get Lean Diet incorporates some of the healthiest eating patterns known to cut the risk of developing diabetes (not to mention heart disease, cancer, and obesity as well). *The reality is that people are more likely to change when they perceive a threat to their children's well-being.*

Maybe for you, SugarDaddy, it will be because our country's latest economic squeeze is already forcing you to move to some greener choices without even realizing it, to ditch things like bottled water, 100-calorie snack packs, and designer coffee drinks in favor of cheaper alternatives such as tap water, conventional snack cartons, and coffee from a pot at home. If so, you will be in the company of millions of Americans who are already feeling a pinch in the pocketbook and making greener buying decisions without even realizing it.[1] *The reality is that people are more likely to change when it's in their own economic best interest.*

As there is a growing call to reinvigorate America through clean energy and green jobs, a cleaner diet offers an immediate, low-tech, and low-cost tool to help us reduce health-care costs. We need fresh ideas that don't depend on costly medical interventions like drugs and surgeries, and a lean and green diet offers a viable alternative.

What's more, in this world of color-coded threats and rapidly changing political and economic conditions, Deborah Madison, author of *The Greens Cookbook,* notes that "knowing that our food is grown nearby and not in some unknown place gives us shoppers a sense of security and connection."[2] This is invaluable to the discomfited American psyche, a "tangible antidote" in the form of local food and increased connection. *The reality is that food provides one of the strongest senses of well-being and security that there is—just ask someone who's gone without it.*

Why will people be moved to change? Because all roads are now pointing to the same place, and it is a crossroad in history on which the very state of the planet hinges. And eating represents an immediate opportunity to make a difference. However you look at it, one thing is clear: The impact of the foods you choose is no longer limited to the immediate impact to your hips or the long-term impact to your health. Your stakes in the food choices you make run deeper than you likely have thought; they run to food companies and agribusiness, to Congress, to Wall Street, to the energy sector, and most important, to the well-being of the planet. And it is the power of your pocketbook, the power you wield every single time you purchase food, that tips those stakes in one clear direction or another. Think of it as good nutrition with a mission.

So this is where we make it happen. And ultimately, the Go Green Get Lean Diet is really pretty simple when you get right down to it; what works for effective weight loss and improved health (strategies I've been using successfully with clients for years) is very, very closely tied with what works for a better planet. Choco-flavored snacks that are fat-free, carb-free, calorie-free, and shrink-wrapped tight enough to survive another Hurricane Katrina may help dieters feel they can "have their cake and eat it too," but it's increasingly clear that that cake is costly to the planet.

As Bill McKibben wrote in his best-selling book *Deep Economy*, it is time for a new way to think about the things we buy, the food we eat, the energy we use, and the power of our pocketbooks. Our purchases can reinforce rather than be at odds with what we value.

This book is about the specific connections between greener eating and better health for you and your family. It seeks to ask the same questions that *you* might pose while standing in the supermarket aisle or at the meat counter, and to outline the benefits to you in terms of weight loss. The goal is to get you to think about your food behavior in the context of being a consumer.

Like many Americans, I am a busy working mother of two young children, and as such, I know firsthand the practical needs and concerns that real life requires as we struggle to "do the right thing." I'm well acquainted with those times when we may be too pooped to experience the *Joy of Cooking* or too tired to engage in the ethical maze of choices confronting us at the supermarket. I also know what it's like to live on a budget with little room to run up a higher food bill in the name of saving the planet. But rest assured, no matter where you are in your life, this book is packed with practical and easy suggestions to make leaner and greener living totally achievable.

My intent is not to highlight yet another dimension of your life about which you should feel guilty yet powerless. If the diet world is any paradigm, using guilt as a motivator creates little, if any, lasting momentum for change. Rather, my goal is to inspire you to create easy, positive changes in your life that will help you look and feel your best. In fact, the framework is surprisingly simple. And unlike other elements of the green movement, from solar panels to hybrids (or a sweaty, overcrowded bus), we all have to engage with food. Daily.

What I hope you will take away from this book is this: Your choices have trade-offs. Always. And for most of us, the mental calculation we do on those trade-offs involves how it impacts us personally in the next 5 minutes. (Think about it: How many people would really down a pint of ice cream at midnight if they were focusing on how they'd feel in the morning? Their brains are humming with the pleasure they want to derive *now*—consequences will be dealt with later.) It's now time to extend that time frame further—to think about what sort of food you want to feed yourself and your children, and what sort of body you want to spend your days in. Here's how it works.

The Go Green Get Lean Diet: A 6-Week Plan for Optimal Eating

The Go Green Get Lean Diet is a 6-week program that tackles one high-carbon area of your diet at a time. At the end of 6 weeks, you will have in place all of the building blocks you need to tread more lightly, literally, for the rest of your life.

Each week will give you a step-by-step road map to making leaner, greener choices. Right now you're in week 1, which will help you see the big picture when it comes to the diet/carbon connection, and all that you have to gain by losing. Here you'll also jump right into action, zeroing in on the top carbon and calorie "hot spots" in your diet, with specific steps to start cooling them.

In week 2, you'll realign one of the most critical elements of your diet, your protein sources, which can potentially help you shed the carbon equivalent of an SUV from your annual carbon footprint and get you on the fast track to lean. In week 2 you'll also be introduced to your new "flexitarian" lifestyle, a lifestyle with a fresh new emphasis on leaner, greener, more sustainable protein sources, enjoying higher-carbon proteins as a once-in-a-while "splurge" instead of daily fare. Red meat, poultry and pork, fish, wild animals—we'll cover them all in week 2 so you have a strong road map to get you and your family on the way to leaner and greener living.

In week 3, you'll begin to work on eating more like a "locavore" a couple of times a week, and you'll discover why lean plates are often green plates. You'll see why eating like a local, while not a catchall for cutting your carbon footprint, is still an important way to boost your nutrition, rediscover flavors and tastes of food, and sow the seeds in your children for a lifetime of healthier eating habits. In week 3 you'll also get the latest skinny on dairy products, another high-carbon component of most people's diets; you'll learn which dairy products are the best choices, and how much you should be getting in order to maximize nutrition and health benefits while keeping this "high-carbon cow" in check.

In week 4, you'll learn how to go for the greener grains, and you'll rediscover ancient grains that have made a comeback to your pantry; these help pack nutrition and flavor into your new lifestyle. It is also time for an ecomakeover for your pantry and fridge; as you complete the Project Pantry Purge, you'll begin to clear away your carbon clutter from your everyday basics. Along the way, you'll discover easy tips for moving from high-carbon, high-calorie, low-nutrition industrial food toward cleaner packaged foods that can give you those valuable shortcuts and time-savers with ingredients and packaging that are greener for the earth and healthier for you. You'll also get an easy, up-to-date primer on fats—and discover how to separate the clean and green from the mean.

In week 5, you'll whittle your waistline and carbon stream even further by redefining what it means to drink responsibly. You'll see which two "Ws" should be in your glass and why, and how to sip sustainably to cut your waste-line *and* your waistline. Then there's also the fun part—we'll take a look at sustainable splurges (things such as coffee, tea, chocolate, and nuts). We'll talk about why it's imperative to make the right choices when it comes to these splurges, as well as why it is important that you splurge in the first place (trust me, it really is important). Throughout the book, you will find stories of people just like you, people who've decided to make the commitment to change and have done so with great success, who share their tips and strategies for making it doable.

In week 6, you will begin the maintenance part of your program. After all, this book is about a new eating style for your new self, not a short-term diet. We'll start with "Your Personal Pep Talk," as if you were to step in my office and meet with me one-on-one. It's a short chapter that reminds you that you alone have the power to create the life, the body, and the state of health that you want for yourself. I want you to read it any time you begin to question the impact of your efforts on your own health and weight, or whenever you waver in your belief in your own potential to be part of the solution of change. It will replace your current "inner monologue" (which, for many people who struggle with weight, is often negative and self-defeating) of stories you tell yourself about why you can't change and how hard it's going to be. Changing that inner monologue is one of the most critical steps in creating lasting success.

In week 6, you'll also find 4 weeks of eating plans, one for each season, that will inspire you with specific, easy, and delicious meal ideas that would easily make up 2 months' worth of eating (with all those leftovers). Many of these recipes, as well as more tips for greener eating, are available at www.leanandgreendiet.com. Still have some lingering questions about the practicality of the plan? Read on to see how easy it can be.

"How Much Weight Will I Lose? Won't I Have to Spend More Cash?"

The Go Green Get Lean Diet is designed as a 6-week program. On average, you can expect to lose about 5 to 9 pounds during the first 2 weeks, with the exact amount depending on how much weight you need to lose and your current eating habits (if you begin this program squarely in the hot zone and you follow all four fixes, you may lose even more). Some of this may be water weight as you focus on clean foods and stop eating all the preservatives and refined carbs that can lead to water retention. Regardless, after just 2 weeks of the Go Green Get Lean Diet, you will no doubt have more energy and be lighter on the scale and in your personal contribution to the global warming crisis.

As you begin the next 4 weeks of the program, the pace of weight loss will then likely slow to about ½ to 2 pounds per week, depending on how much weight you have to lose. Losing weight any faster can mean a loss of metabolism-boosting lean muscle and increased hunger and fatigue. And there's nothing sustainable about that! As each week addresses specific areas of your diet that are critical to lean and green living, the exact amount will also depend on how quickly you read through and complete each step of the program and adopt the lean and green lifestyle.

The other thing you will notice changing is *where* your food dollar is going. Let me be clear: You do not need to spend more to eat better. It just takes moving from your current comfort zone of eating habits (which often comes with comfy sweats) to one of being a proactive steward of your planet and your body. You will be changing your spending habits to be a more conscious consumer. Dollars that stop going to dirty areas of your diet will then be freed up to help you build a fresher, delicious, fun, and sustainable plate.

Once you redefine the notion of "splurge," it's easy to recognize and celebrate the joy that comes from eating in a way that is naturally delicious and served *without* the heaping side order of planetary guilt. Best of all, you can still include your favorite treats from time to time (and you will likely discover new ones along the way).

"Should I Take Any Vitamins or Supplements?"

"Food first" is definitely the gold standard when it comes to better health. In other words, chasing that fast-food meal with supplements does not "even out" poor dietary choices. However, a standard daily multivitamin (it doesn't have to be a fancy brand) containing nearly 100 percent of the RDA for most nutrients is likely a good insurance policy. (I say "most nutrients" because some nutrients, such as calcium, are simply too large to be included in a single pill, and fat-soluble vitamins such as A and K are often included in lesser levels.) Be sure to choose one that's right for your gender and age (and if you are pregnant or planning to become pregnant, choose a prenatal vitamin with your health practitioner).

In addition, if you are at risk for osteoporosis or do not consume enough calcium-containing foods, consider a calcium supplement; adults over age 50 need 1,200 milligrams per day, while adults under 50 need 1,000 milligrams per day. Choose one made from calcium citrate or calcium carbonate that delivers 500 to 600 milligrams in each dose. Take this twice a day to maximize absorption. Look for one that also has vitamin D. In addition to boosting calcium absorption, it may protect you against disease. The research on vitamin D continues to expand and show health benefits, and it seems that many Americans (especially older Americans) are deficient.

Lastly, if you don't eat fish, consider an omega-3 supplement. Look for a supplement that provides 1,000 milligrams each day of omega-3s in the form of EPA and DHA for maximum heart benefits. Read the label, because you may need to take two in order to reach this amount. (For example, a 1,000-milligram capsule may contain 250 milligrams of EPA and 250 milligrams of DHA, which adds up to 500 milligrams of omega-3 fat, so you would need to take two.)

And remember, you are what you eat. Those words are as true today as they were a million years ago when some rather smart person first uttered them. *You are what you eat.* Take it in. Live it. Breathe it. And eat it.

Are you ready to jump in with me? Fantastic. Let's start cooling the planet together. It's time to tackle some of your biggest hot spots and get you on the fast track to lightening up.

It *Is* Easy Being Green: Four Quick Shortcuts to Cut Your Carbon Footprint without Touching Your Diet

If you're starting to feel concerned about how much your diet may need to change in order to lighten your carbon load, take heart: *Some of the biggest pieces of your "food footprint" come from your food-related* **behaviors** *rather than your actual food choices.* Even if you change nothing, zilch, nada about what's on your plate, here are four quick shortcuts to take a big bite out of your diet's carbon footprint without even touching your diet.

1. **Become a sustainable shopper.** Your individual behavior as a shopper is quite possibly the biggest issue in determining the total carbon footprint of your food. In our suburban culture, we are logging more miles than ever before on food. How often do you shop? How many stores do you visit to save money? What type of bags do you use? Your habits as a shopper matter.

2. **Cut your waste-line.** A recent British study concluded that, on average, Brits waste about 30 percent of food they buy, and that they "could make carbon savings equivalent to taking an estimated 1 in 5 cars off the road if we avoided throwing away all the food that we could have eaten."[3] In our economic downturn, I imagine few Americans can afford to toss one in three grocery bags, but my hunch is we're not too far off from our English friends, probably without realizing it. Whether it's tossing out leftovers or buying a cookie at the mall and then guiltily throwing it away after three bites, the energy involved in growing and transporting that food has been wasted. And, as food decays in landfills, it emits one of the most potent warming gases of all—methane.

3. **Reduce, reuse, reuse, reuse some more . . . then recycle.** It's easy to get bogged down in questions such as "Should I buy aluminum or plastic? Frozen or fresh?" But one thing is clear; it is what happens to the food packaging *after* you're done that is critical in determining the actual carbon footprint of that choice. While the idea of "reusing" often gets glossed over in this oft-quoted trio of action steps, it's critical to cutting your carbon footprint.

4. **Make sure your appliances are energy efficient.** Ho hum, sounds boring, right? Wrong. A striking conclusion made by the University of California, Davis, Sustainability

Institute after an extensive review of the literature was this: One of the biggest "hot spots" in determining a person's personal "food footprint" is that household food storage and preparation account for 25 to 30 percent of the total carbon load of that food.[4] So tucking those organic farmers' market strawberries into a 20-year-old fridge that's belching out warming gases misses the point.

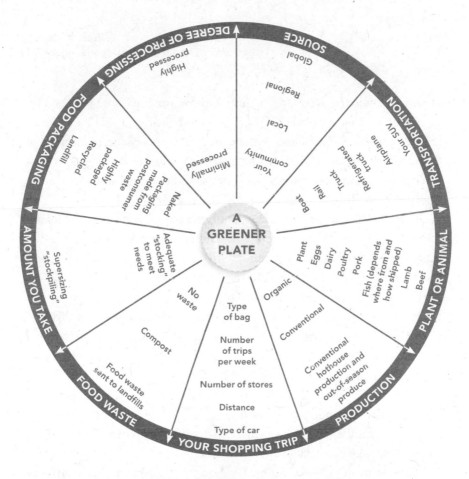

"How Do I Join the Green Plate Club?"
There are many factors that impact your food's carbon footprint. While there are certainly exceptions, this wheel can be used as a handy tool to help you see how green your plate really is.

CHAPTER 3

GET STARTED NOW

Get on the Fast Track to Lean and Green

"Despite the appearance of an endless bounty of food, it is a fragile bounty, dependent upon the integrity of the global oil production, refining, and delivery system."

—William Church,
"Why Our Food Is So Dependent on Oil"

When it comes to carbon footprints, Americans have some of the biggest feet in the world. How big? A recent study by MIT students found that even a homeless American still has a carbon footprint of 8.5 tons—*twice* the global average. And his shelter-living peers produce a whopping 20 tons of CO_2 per capita. What uses the most energy in our lifestyle? Transportation, housing, and food.[1]

The Go Green Get Lean Diet is about to take you on a delicious journey that will reconnect you with the right types of foods that can make you healthy and trimmer while also thinning your carbon footprint at the same time. These are foods that are fresh and flavorful, that are connected to a sense of place and transport you away from all the faux food that is oozing from every corner of our culture today. It's food that can absolutely be enjoyed in a way that allows you to thrive, but doesn't compromise the ability of those who come after you to do the same thing.

As it stands now, so much of our current eating landscape dulls these vibrant connections—we are encouraged to gobble down our food while multitasking, and our children are learning that dinner comes from the car rather than the kitchen.

Earlier in my career, when I was actively counseling clients, I could already see the outcome of this lifestyle. One-third of my practice was comprised of young adults who came to me because they were living on their own for the first time, with no idea of how to cook or plan meals and shopping lists. All they knew how to do was survive on takeout. And they were miserable and often gaining weight.

That's why week 1, the "Take Action" phase, of the Go Green Get Lean Diet is designed to address the biggest problems associated with our food system, and the payback, in terms of both weight loss and a lightened carbon footprint, is going to be huge. Specifically, it's going to do three things:

- Tackle some of the largest contributors to your personal carbon food footprint each day

- Eliminate the overprocessed, overpackaged, oversized, nutritionally empty foods that are currently hogging up space in your fridge, pantry, and daily food jaunts

- Replace these with sustainable, fresh, whole, delicious foods that are much healthier for you and the planet

If you do nothing but read this chapter and put these quick fixes into action, you'll have cooled some of the largest areas of your food's carbon footprint and cleared out a bunch of unnecessary calories that are keeping you from moving toward your personal best health. Done. Enough said. Close the book. But if you want to know the answer to the "whys" behind it, or want to delve deeper into the new green and lean cuisine, keep reading.

"Can My Eating Habits Really Be Warming the Planet?"

Yes, and it is happening quicker than we thought.

As I've said, the consequences of your daily food choices go well beyond whether or not you'll be able to fit into your "skinny jeans" tomorrow. Your choices resonate high up into the atmosphere, and like the extra fat cells on your derriere, they'll linger there for a long time unless you do something about them. According to a 2008 report in *Human Ecology,* our food supply now accounts for about 19 percent of total US greenhouse gas emissions.[2] And researchers estimate that up to 50 percent of this "energy bill" could be trimmed with a few tweaks to the American diet (hint:

eat less animal products and junk food, and eat more local food) and a few changes in packaging and agriculture.

Here's the deal. To lose weight, you have to change what you eat. You need to eat less "junk" and more real food. To cut your personal carbon footprint, you need to change what you eat. You need to concentrate on eating less "junk" and more real food. See any overlap? Wonderful.

So let's get started.

COOL HOT SPOT #1:
SKIP BEEF AND CHEESE FOR 2 WEEKS

A key hallmark of an SUV diet is the amount of beef you consume. A 2006 UN report found livestock production (especially beef) created almost 20 percent of total greenhouse gases worldwide, eclipsing even transportation. A 2008 report in *Environmental Science and Technology* estimated that red meat (30 percent) and dairy (18 percent) account for nearly half of all greenhouse gases from food in an average US household. This is why skipping beef and cheese is Quick Fix #1. No other food is likely to have as significant an impact on your dietary carbon footprint as beef. Cheese is also eliminated in this phase because it is another high-carbon, high-calorie food, especially if it comes from cows. Remember, we're certainly not taking it away for good—we're just shelving it until we see how to make greener choices. Want another compelling reason? It's also an easy way to a leaner diet.

LEAN BENEFITS

Realigning the amount of beef and cheese in your diet does two things: It helps trim excess calories from unhealthy saturated fat from your diet (and thus your waistline), and it can reduce damage to your arteries. That's because cheese and beef represent the top two sources of artery-clogging saturated fat in the American diet, accounting for 13.1 percent and 11.7 percent respectively.[3] And Americans are consuming more cheese than ever. According to the USDA's Economic Research Service, between 1970 and 2005, the availability of cheese nearly tripled, from 11 pounds per person to a heart-stopping 31 pounds per person. Ounce for ounce, most cuts of beef (such as a burger, ribs, or steak) are higher in calories than fish or poultry. As a general rule, replacing beef with fish, poultry, or wild game (i.e., venison), you will cut unhealthy saturated fat while trimming calories from your plate.

While many beef cuts come in a high-calorie package, cheese almost always comes that way, weighing in at about 100 calories an ounce (much of it in the form of saturated fat). (Here's a news flash: To lose weight, it is best to omit any food that packs 100 calories per ounce.) Even low-fat and fat-free cheeses are still high carbon, so for now, during your "Take Action" phase, avoid them.

So what should you eat? For the next 2 weeks, swap all of your beef meals for vegetarian ones (without cheese). This swap immediately moves you to the coolest place to eat from a global warming standpoint, and points you to the leanest choices as well.

Here are some easy ways to accomplish this: Order a grilled veggie and hummus sandwich instead of a cheeseburger, make bean burritos instead of beef ones, and enjoy a warming bowl of oatmeal instead of a meat and-cheese omelet. Total savings in 1 day? Almost 9 pounds of carbon and 890 calories. Do this every day for 2 weeks and those savings multiply to become 122 pounds of carbon (about 6 gallons of gasoline) and 12,460 calories (3.5 pounds). Now think if your whole family did it. Your friends.

Check out the "Is Your Diet Warming the Planet?" table on page 33 to see the immediate savings you'll make with each meal. Don't worry, though; omitting beef and cheese entirely from your diet is only for 2 weeks, at which point you can begin reintroducing the *right* kinds of beef and cheese in the *right* quantities to maximize health.

As you move through your program, you'll see that each chapter will begin with a "Prescription" that provides specific guidelines on how much of a given food you should include each week or month. But the actual portion size you choose at each meal is up to you. Take chicken, for example; essentially, you can enjoy up to 12 ounces of chicken per week. I suggest three 4-ounce servings over the course of the week as a general guideline on "how," but it's important for you to work within your own comfort zone. Do you like the feeling of "meat on the plate" at nearly every dinner meal? Then serve smaller sizes more often (3 ounces of meat is roughly the size of a deck of cards), and heap lots of seasonal vegetables, beans, and whole grains alongside it. Or you could toss 2 ounces of chopped grilled chicken (about the size of two matchbooks) into your salad 6 days of the week. Alternately, you could skip the bird all week and then enjoy an 8-ounce grilled chicken breast at the Saturday barbecue and sneak some leftovers for a yummy sandwich the next day, tucking in 4 ounces' worth.

It's the same logic with pork and lamb; you can savor one large sitting of pork tenderloin, or else make it last by tucking 3 ounces of sliced pork loin into a veggie stir-fry one night, and another night stuffing peppers or zucchini with a mixture that includes 2 ounces of ground lamb along with rice, mint, currants, and pine nuts. Indeed, "stretching" meat to go further by pairing it with plant-based cuisine not only has economic benefits, but it also is one of the hallmarks of some of the world's healthiest (and most delicious) eating styles, such as the Mediterranean diet.

But we're getting ahead of ourselves. Let's focus on how eliminating beef and dairy from your diet can impact the planet, too.

GREEN BENEFITS

Calorie for calorie, growing plants is a much more efficient use of "fuel" than raising animals; growing produce (fruits and vegetables) requires about 2 fossil fuel calories to create 1 calorie of food, while growing animal protein requires 20 to 80 fossil fuel calories to create 1 food calorie.[4] And research from both the United States and the Netherlands has found that beef and dairy account for about 50 percent of a household's food footprint.[5]

Taking this oil-dependent staple off of your plate for 2 weeks creates immediate savings. Now let's look at another way we could save; consider that in 2000 Americans grilled up an annual average of 113 pounds of beef per person, at an average of 2.17 pounds (boneless and trimmed) per week.[6] This translates into about 2,430 food calories per week (assuming lean cuts of beef at about 70 calories per ounce). Look at those calories in terms of the fuel calories required to bring them to your plate, and Quick Fix #1 cuts at least 100,000 fossil fuel calories from your lifestyle in those first 2 weeks. Imagine if each household in America did this; if everyone lowered their beef consumption by 4 pounds over the course of 1 year, it would save 1 trillion gallons of water, which is the volume that flows over Niagara Falls for 20 consecutive days.[7]

IS YOUR DIET WARMING THE PLANET?[8]

Check out these immediate carbon and calorie savings that can be achieved through leaner living. The Bon Appétit Management Company is one of the leaders in sustainable eating with their Low Carbon Diet Initiative. Using data from 40 peer-reviewed studies that looked at total life cycle and carbon, they have created a helpful online calculator that lets you see the immediate carbon savings of making greener swaps. I've also added the calorie savings so you can see why it's usually a leaner bet, too.

INSTEAD OF THIS	EAT THIS	AND SAVE THIS
Beef soft tacos (2), 4 lbs CO_2e, 490 calories	Black bean soft tacos (2), 1 lb CO_2e, 260 calories	3 lbs CO_2e, 230 calories
Grilled cheese sandwich, 1.9 lbs CO_2e, 319 calories	Grilled veggie and hummus sandwich, 0.6 lb CO_2e, 306 calories	1.3 lbs CO_2e, 13 calories
Cheeseburger, 4 lbs CO_2e, 572 calories	Grilled chicken sandwich, 1.5 lbs CO_2e, 361 calories	2.5 lbs CO_2e, 211 calories
Meat and cheese omelet, 3.3 lbs CO_2e, 562 calories	Steel-cut oats with yogurt and fruit, 1 lb CO_2e, 168 calories	2.3 lbs CO_2e, 394 calories

TAKE ACTION NOW

- Swap all your beef and cheese choices in the next 2 weeks for vegetarian ones. Choose from one of the recipes in the back of this book or one of the thousands of free online vegetarian recipes, open a favorite cookbook, or ask friends and family members for their favorite vegetarian meal ideas. Ounce for ounce, beans, legumes, and tofu shave significant calories and fat from your plate while boosting fiber and phyto-nutrients when used instead of beef and cheese choices (see "Focus on the Food Chain" to save calories, carbon, and cost starting on page 53).

- Move any beef you currently have into your freezer, and cross it off of your shopping list for now. Your cheese should last in the fridge. If not, give it away.

- Log onto www.eatlowcarbon.org to calculate the carbon footprint of the foods you commonly eat.

COOL HOT SPOT #2:
START SNACKING SUSTAINABLY

Smokestacks, automobiles, private planes . . . and gummy bears? Does what you nibble in the minivan while waiting for soccer practice to end, or that treat you purloin from the office candy jar, really have that big of an impact?

Yes indeed, and here's why: More than 80 percent of Americans snack, and experts estimate that, overall, snacks contribute about 23 percent of total calories to a person's diet. This is why your snack habits play a significant role in your weight and health. It's also why your snacks probably play a bigger role in the carbon footprint of your diet than you may think.

In a nutshell, snacks can do one of two things. When done correctly, snacking can keep your energy level up and your blood sugar stable; it can prevent you from overeating at night; and it can deliver key nutrients, all while keeping you in a cool shade of green. On the flip side, snacking can pack on pounds, zap energy, and contribute to carbon bloat. It all depends on what you're noshing.

LEAN BENEFITS

Americans currently consume about 500 more calories a day than they did back in the 1970s (which goes a long way to explain why Americans *weigh* more than they did in the 1970s).[9] Why? We are surrounded by more food, more of the time, than ever before. Supersize portions and eating opportunities beckon constantly. Essentially, we have created a culture where the line between "eating" and "not eating" has been obscured, so that most of us are either sipping or nibbling something most of the day.

Then there is the issue of the quality of most snacks themselves. How do I say this gently? Most snack foods today, especially those marketed for optimal convenience, are of dubious quality. Highly processed foods contain a long list of ingredients that sound like they came from a lab and provide little real nutrition. Perhaps the snack comes fortified with a smattering of nutrients to give it a healthier image, but still you're better off with real, whole food rather than what I call food product. And some of today's "snacks" pack a caloric punch more suited for someone who's about to chop wood for an hour rather than, say, plop their rear into a chair and surf the Web researching wood prices for a home remodel.

Further, when it comes to snacking, the research is clear. When people are surrounded by large amounts of ready-to-eat foods, they eat more.[10] *In other words, overly convenient foods boost calorie intake.* It also turns out that for people trying to lose weight, they may be better off shunning the 100-calorie snack packs. A 2008 study in the *Journal of Consumer Research* found that people ate nearly twice as much from 100-calorie snack packs than did people who were given larger packages.[11] Another drawback was that people viewed "diet-friendly" packages as a sort of calorie-free ride and ate more than those who were given regular-size packages. Believe me, a lot of research has gone into how to make it possible for you to reach for snacks whenever and wherever the impulse strikes you. To give just one example, consider the emergence of all of these "bites," such as cheesecake or ice cream, that have pushed what was once considered special occasion splurges into the realm of a bona fide daily snack option. While it may be good for food companies' bottom lines, it's terrible for your own bottom.

Making a shift to cleaner snacks is Quick Fix #2 because it immediately packs more nutrition and fewer calories into your snacks while reducing carbon and saving money. And you will become refreshed and rebalanced after taking a break from all of those overly salted, sugary food products.

So how often should you snack? As a rough guideline, most people

A SIMPLE WAY TO DOUBLE YOUR WEIGHT LOSS: KEEP A FOOD JOURNAL

Not a jogger? Forget shelling out big bucks for diet foods and fancy weight loss programs, and consider trying the other proven diet tactic that begins with "j"—journaling. A 2008 study by Kaiser Permanente found that those who kept a food log lost twice as much weight as those who didn't.[12]

Accountability to yourself is a powerful thing, and a journal helps you see your own eating patterns—the good, the bad, and the ugly. For many of my clients, it was a key in producing an "aha" moment that motivated them to change.

It also prevents what I call "eating amnesia," making you focus more closely on the portion sizes and "freebies" that can sneak into your day. Best of all, it's easy and free. Leverage these powerful benefits to your advantage and start tracking. A few moments of planning can yield tremendous reward. Athletes do it. Financial planners do it. And you should do it. It's a key to getting the results that you want.

Simple Tips for Keeping a Food Journal

Go high tech or low tech, but go. Use whatever method of tracking works for you—whether that's a simple piece of paper, an e-mail or text message to yourself, or a PDA program—but *the key is to start tracking*. Keep a food

need to refuel every 3 to 4 hours to stay energized and satisfied. This usually translates into a midmorning and midafternoon snack, each about 100 to 175 calories. Eat too little, and it might not do the trick, while snacks creeping up toward 250 calories start to resemble a meal. Think airline portions (back when airlines actually gave you food, that is). If you find you prefer to snack less than this and can still meet your goals, that's okay, too.

What should you choose? Start with any snack listed in "Your Guide to Sustainable Snacking" on page 40. The keys to sustainable snacking are actually pretty easy to remember. For your waistline, keep the calories in the right range (which we've already defined journal for at least a week of what you eat, including how much of each item. If you can spare a bit more time, include the time of day, where you are, and how you feel. You can make your own food journal, or print out a free form at www.leanandgreendiet.com.

Write as you go. After each meal or snack, quickly jot down what you ate. Keep your food journal in a spot that's handy for you, whether that's the kitchen, on your desk, or in your purse; saving up for the end of the day may raise the odds of forgetting something and make it suddenly seem more time-consuming.

Be specific. Estimate specific portion sizes, whether in cups, ounces, or "how many" (e.g., 1 cup of pasta, 12-ounce latte, four cookies). This will help you see precisely how much you're eating and is the reason why a journal is so insightful for most people.

Include the good, the bad, and the ugly. This isn't about just keeping track of the "good" stuff you're proud to show someone else. Include all of your food and drinks, even those consumed during weekends, late nights, or anything in between. For most people, there is a big difference in weekdays versus weekends, and you need to understand your own variations in order to make positive changes.

Show me yours, I'll show you mine. For even more powerful results, show someone else your food journal and tell the person what you've learned. The extra accountability makes you even more likely to stick to your leaner, greener guns and get losing.

above). For your carbon footprint and your health, snacks should be real food (minimally processed, all-natural foods, preferably something in season). And, for maximum staying power and energy, choose a snack that includes some protein or heart-healthy fats.

GREEN BENEFITS

There is an immense discrepancy between the amount of fossil fuel our highly processed, convenience-oriented snacks are hogging, versus the limited nutrition or health benefits they provide (and in some cases, the very real diseases they help foster, such as high blood pressure, heart disease, or high insulin response). Let's think of snacks, for a moment, in the context of resource use.

Did you know that it takes about 98 tons (a staggering 196,000 pounds) of prehistoric buried plant material to produce just 1 gallon of gasoline?[13] A 2003 study from the University of Utah determined that you would have to put the equivalent of 40 acres' worth of wheat into the tank of your car for every 20 miles you drive. For most people's SUVs, that equates to less than 1 gallon of gasoline. Forty acres of wheat to create less than 1 gallon of gasoline! How many acres of wheat went into meeting your snack attack?

"Every day, people are using the fossil fuel equivalent of all plant matter that grows on the Earth in an entire year," the researchers wrote. (Of note: They also included right down to microscopic ocean life.) Yes, and in America, they're blowing through it on essential life staples such as cheesy doodads and calorie-dense bars made with choco-bits and fats specially engineered to cruise through unabsorbed so we can eat them guilt free.

So to recap: It takes millions of years to create the biomass that becomes crude oil that then becomes gasoline that is used to create a snack that takes less than 2 minutes to eat. Hmmm . . . does that seem sustainable? And are humans really designed to handle eating 300-calorie "snacks," often devoid of true nutrition? Of course not. This type of eating is not sustainable for anyone, except, perhaps, food companies.

Look back at "How Much Fossil Fuel Did Your Lunch Require?" on page 6 for a moment and consider the journey required to produce something like a 100-calorie snack pack, something so easily scarfed down in just a few minutes, something that provides no specific

---

CO_2 AND CO_2 EQUIVALENTS

Carbon Dioxide Equivalents (or CO_2e) is an internationally accepted standard of measure that considers the total impact of all global warming gases (including methane and nitrous oxide) from a particular choice.

nutritional advantage when compared to real food. Biomass aside, for each gallon of gasoline needed to produce and get that snack into your mouth (which we've already covered), nearly 19 pounds of carbon have been released into the atmosphere. Yikes.

The more types of highly processed food products like this that you eat, the greater the percentage of your total food calories that are likely creating carbon bloat, not to mention belly bloat. Plus, in my experience, consuming these products may well leave you feeling less satisfied and energized. (Doesn't that defeat the whole point of snacking in the first place?)

So what does that mean for the way we snack? Fortunately, there are tons of delicious, easy noshes that are convenient, fast, fresh, and tasty, as well as a lot better for your weight and the planet. It's pretty simple; snack on real food rather than "food product." See pages 40 and 41 for a great list.

TAKE ACTION NOW

Eliminate all of those 100-calorie snack packs, single-serving-size packages, and any snacks that have high-fructose corn syrup in the ingredient list. Clear away your carbon clutter by donating these high-carbon snacks to a food pantry, a school, a church group, or some other organization. Instead of snacking on produce flown in from another country, buy fruits and vegetables that are local to you and in season as much as possible (if you're starting your program in the winter, this may be a bit more difficult; see Chapter 9 for a guide to seasonal produce in your area).

COOL HOT SPOT #3:
SKIP THE ADDED SUGARS, ARTIFICIAL SWEETENERS, AND ALCOHOL FOR 2 WEEKS

"Hold on a minute here. In the last chapter you assured me you weren't one of those nagging nutritionists pulling every pleasure from my plate. But this is starting to sound suspiciously like that's exactly what you're up to."

Okay, fair comment. So let me assure you that this isn't a

(continued on page 42)

YOUR GUIDE TO SUSTAINABLE SNACKING

Sustainable snacking is one change that will serve you (and the planet) well in the long haul. The route to fabulous snacks starts with fabulous food. Consider this a starting point, but by all means feel free to experiment with the best that the seasons (and your geography) have to offer. All snacks listed below contain 100 to 175 calories. Be sure to avoid any with cheese until after your 2-week turnaround phase.

THE STANDARDS

100–175 Calories:

- 10 kalamata olives (106 cal)
- ½ cup shelled steamed or boiled edamame (100 cal)
- ¾ cup edamame in pods with a pinch of sea salt (135 cal)
- 1 oz almonds, peanuts, or pistachios (dry roasted and/or minimally salted if high blood pressure is not a concern) (164 cal)
- ¼ cup Healthy Trail Mix (146 cal) (see page 282)
- ½ cup pumpkin seeds (143 cal)
- 1 oz sunflower seeds (165 cal)
- 3 Tbsp roasted soybeans (152 cal)
- 1 Tbsp almond butter on ½ slice of whole grain bread or 2 whole wheat crackers (120 cal)
- 1 Tbsp cashew butter spread on 1 cup of apple slices or on ½ medium banana (143 cal)
- 3 cups air-popped popcorn (134 cal)
- 1 Tbsp peanut butter with 1 cup raw carrot and celery sticks (130 cal)
- 6 oz fat-free organic yogurt and ½ cup fresh blueberries (140 cal)
- ½ cup organic fat-free Greek yogurt drizzled with 2 tsp raw honey and 1 Tbsp slivered almonds (142 cal)
- ⅓ cup baba ghannouj (eggplant dip) with 1 oz local whole wheat bread, naan, or pita (170 cal)
- ⅓ cup Garlicky Edamame Hummus (see page 241) with ½ cup crudités (175 cal)
- 6" whole wheat tortilla with ¼ cup black beans and 2 Tbsp fresh salsa (140 cal)
- 1 hard-cooked egg mashed with 1 tsp extra virgin olive oil on ½ slice dark rye bread (158 cal)

SUMMER FIX

100 Calories or Fewer:

1 fresh cantaloupe wedge or 1 fresh fig wrapped with 1 thin slice real prosciutto (70 cal)

A 100 percent frozen fruit bar or 3 frozen cubes of 100 percent pomegranate, blueberry, or cherry juice (70 cal)

½ cup confetti bell pepper strips (any combo of red, yellow, orange, or green peppers) dipped in 2 Tbsp Tuscan Lemon Vinaigrette (see page 239) or hummus (95 cal)

1 cup cubed watermelon or honeydew with ¼ cup organic fat-free cottage cheese (100 cal)

101–175 Calories:

⅓ cup sliced fresh figs with 2 Tbsp real ricotta on 2 Wasa crisps (or use 2 tsp fig jam in winter) (160 cal)

2 Tbsp olive tapenade tossed with ½ cup sliced cherry tomatoes on 4 whole grain crackers (126 cal)

½ cup Summer Pepper Sauté (sauté a variety of bell peppers with 1 tsp olive oil, garlic, and a pinch of kosher salt; add fresh chopped basil at the end) served with 1 oz pita crisps (164 cal)

WINTER WARM-UPS

95–175 Calories:

Handful of dried local fruit (e.g., cherries, cranberries, blueberries, or raisins) and ½ oz dark chocolate (142 cal)

10 dark chocolate chips and 10 walnut halves (168 cal)

1 cup organic local fat-free milk (or soymilk), steamed, with 1 tsp almond extract and 1 Tbsp dark cocoa powder (114 cal)

¼ cup avocado "mash" (with 1 Tbsp fresh lime or orange juice and a pinch of kosher salt) on ½ slice whole grain bread (138 cal)

⅓ cup chickpeas or cooked lentils swirled with 2 Tbsp pesto, salsa verde, tapenade, or other intensely flavored spread (175 cal)

Citrus/avocado bowl: ½ cup grapefruit or orange wedges with 2 slices of avocado, cubed, tossed lightly with a pinch of sea salt (95 cal)

Broiled grapefruit with a dollop of fat-free yogurt and sprinkled with cinnamon or star anise (100 cal)

Reference: The Food Processor, ESHA version 8.8, December 2006
USDA CALCULATOR: http://www.nal.usda.gov/fnic/foodcomp/search/index.html
(Accessed July 8, 2008)

permanent removal as much as a way to help rebalance and reset your palate and your cravings, particularly those nasty ones you haven't been able to tame.

For most people, the reality is "the more you eat, the more you crave." Eliminating added sugars and sweeteners is one of the fastest ways to free your body of chronic sugar cravings. Over and over again I have seen clients so wrapped up in a sweetness seesaw that when they lay off of it for 2 weeks, they have a clarity of energy (and often weight loss) that sparks their enthusiasm for more satisfying and sustainable snacks to meet their health and weight goals. And here's some more good news: You've already *done* much of this heavy lifting by switching to sustainable snacks.

Getting rid of the sweet stuff will also help slow your carbon burn, as these ingredients are often found in high-carbon, highly processed foods such as soft drinks, energy drinks, juice "blends," and desserts. Remember, it's only for 2 weeks. After your body has "reprogrammed" itself, you can start bringing the right kinds of green treats back into your life.

LEAN BENEFITS

You'll notice this Quick Fix specifies that we want to avoid *added* sugars. That is because naturally occurring sugars present in foods such as fruits, vegetables, dairy products, and grains are healthy and perfectly fine to keep enjoying in your diet; in fact, these foods will be a cornerstone of your new lean and green lifestyle. (During the height of the low-carb craze, when clients would tell me they were avoiding things such as bananas and carrots and apples because "they were loaded with sugar," I would respond like this: "Let me ask you something; do you believe the reason Americans are the fattest people on the planet is because we're eating too many bananas, carrots, and apples?") Naturally occurring sugars found in whole foods like these provide energy and sweetness without the dark underbelly of blood sugar swings and cravings.

Added sugars and sweeteners themselves aren't so much the problem, but rather it's the massive amounts that most Americans are eating. On average, Americans indulge in about 150 pounds of sugar per person each year, which is about 31 teaspoons of sugar per day, or about 500 extra calories a day from sugar.[14] This means that most of us are getting more sugar in one day than our hunter-gatherer ancestors consumed *in their entire lifetimes.*

Roughly half of this amount is in the form of high-fructose corn syrup (HFCS), a highly refined corn sweetener that is prevalent in nearly all processed food. For manufacturers, the benefits of HFCS are clear. It's cheap, it's plentiful, and it is shelf-stable into the next millennium (consider that our food supply provides about 200 calories per person each day in soft drinks alone, all in the form of HFCS).

While HFCS is certainly not the sole cause of our obesity crisis, it definitely plays a role; between 1970 and 1990, consumption of HFCS increased by more than *1,000 percent* (that is not a typo).[15] During that same period, there has been a suspiciously similar rise in obesity rates; between 1970 and 2000, obesity rates more than doubled, from 15 percent to more than 30 percent of the adult population. And worse, obesity among children ages 12 to 19 more than tripled, climbing from 4.2 percent to 15.3 percent. Further, a 2004 study that followed 50,000 nurses found that those who drank one soda or fruit drink per day (containing either HFCS or sugar) had an 80 percent increased risk of developing type 2 diabetes and were more likely to gain weight.[16]

We'll talk more about artificial sweeteners in Chapter 14 when we discuss diet sodas, but the reason artificial sweeteners are also included in this list is that they still can promote a craving for sweetness, and they are highly processed (which means high-carbon) ingredients found in high-carbon food products (as opposed to real food, which is what you want to be eating more of). And while you may assume that foods containing zero-calorie sweeteners get you on the fast track to weight loss, think again; the research has found that they may actually make it *harder* to lose weight.[17] (Or if you want to take a less scientific approach, simply ask yourself this: If all of these products *worked,* shouldn't it stand to reason that people using them would be thinner? Then take a good look around.)

As for alcohol and its role in weight loss or gain, it's important to remember that alcohol is almost twice as high in calories as carbohydrates, weighing in at 7 calories per gram as opposed to carbohydrates' 4 calories per gram. And, because your body will burn calories from alcohol for energy first, before calories from carbohydrate or fat, you can see why it's easy to pack on the pounds if you consume alcohol regularly.

An analogy my clients always seemed to love is equating drinks with bread. Consider that one alcoholic drink has about 130 to 150 calories, significantly more than a regular slice of bread (which contains about 100 calories per slice). So if you normally have one glass of alcohol a night, for example, that's like having, oh, an extra loaf of bread a week. Should you be eating an extra loaf of bread a week if your goal is to become a lean and green machine? My professional answer would be no. If you drink, ahem, say just a tad more than that, the savings when you stop will be even bigger.

The other reason I advise clients to remove alcohol for the first 2 weeks is that because drinking alcohol can lower your inhibitions (in case you haven't heard), it can derail even the most well-intentioned eaters when they're just starting out on a new eating style. In some people, alcohol may also stimulate appetite, so for these reasons, it's better to eliminate it for the first 2 weeks. The added bonus? An immense psychological boost to your commitment to health and a new you from the added weight loss that this provides.

Unlike many other eating plans, where alcohol is *verboten* the entire time you're on the plan, you can resume drinking wine in moderation as part of a delicious lean and green cuisine after 2 weeks. If you're not trying to lose weight but simply looking to green your diet, then feel free to continue to enjoy a bit of wine in moderation now.

GREEN BENEFITS

"Sweeteners and sugars" is a broad category indeed—there are beet and cane sugars; then there is HFCS, which comes from refining corn; then there are the artificial sweeteners. So to keep it simple, let's focus on the key characteristics that make them high-carbon choices when compared to the naturally occurring sugars found in whole foods.

While there is little specific data in the United States about the carbon footprint of any of these sweeteners per se, a 2007 industry report identified the key factors of the UK beet sugar carbon footprint as the following:[18]

Beet Cultivation: 14–26 percent

Refining: 47–58 percent

Packing and Transportation: 9–11 percent

Waste Recycling and Disposal: 4–6 percent

You can quickly see that the single largest element of carbon footprint is the refining step, which isn't surprising. Take a basic food found in nature, and if you start processing it highly, it's going to add pounds of carbon to that food's final footprint. (I am going to make the same assumption for the leap from corn to high-fructose corn syrup, knowing the large number of refining steps involved.) Artificial sweeteners, on the other hand, being synthesized in a factory (from other ingredients, each of which has its own carbon footprint) before they even get sent for use in foods and beverages, are high-carbon little buggers from the start.

Perhaps it's little coincidence, then, that both sugars and sweeteners are often key ingredients in highly processed foods, adding layer upon layer of petroleum and carbon to each step, whether it's in a candy bar, a sugary coffee drink, or a cookie purchased from under a glowing heat lamp. Or perhaps teaspoon-size amounts of that sweetener are wrapped in individual packages and sent to coffee shops around the country.

So what's the green impact? Researchers estimate it requires nearly 10,000 fossil fuel calories to produce 1 pound of sugar, or about ⅓ of a gallon of gasoline.[19] If every American cut out those 31 teaspoons of daily sugar for 2 weeks, this one change would spare roughly 90 million pounds of CO_2 from entering the atmosphere.

Here's another thought. The HFCS in one 32-ounce soda requires about ⅓ of a pound of corn to produce.[20] If every American cut out just one 32-ounce soda per week, that's 100 million pounds of corn—enough to feed a meal to every starving person in Africa. And in the process, each American would easily shed those pesky "last 10 pounds."

Of course, I will be the first to agree that sugars bring flavor to other foods, can add delicious taste to any eating plan, and can be enjoyed as part of a leaner, greener lifestyle for most healthy individuals. I'm certainly not saying we should never eat it. In fact, after just 2 weeks, you'll be able to reintroduce things such as honey, maple syrup, and small amounts of regular, old-fashioned sugar. However, we currently consume way too much sugar, and for many of my clients, eating too much sugar fuels an unhealthy drive to seek more, adding "empty calories" to their diets and pounds to their carbon footprint. So experience the clarity and energy that come from skipping it for 2 weeks; then you can introduce smaller portions of green treats that are more sustainable for you *and* the planet.

TAKE ACTION NOW

- Enjoy all of the *naturally* occurring sugars that the whole foods in your diet provide, such as those found in fruit, vegetables, beans, dairy products, and whole grains.

- Read ingredient labels on food packaging and avoid anything with the following: high-fructose corn syrup, corn syrup, sucrose, maltose, dextrose, fructose, galactose, sugar, fruit concentrate, or barley malt. For now, also skip the natural sugars such as honey, molasses, and maple syrup.

- Hold (for now) any sweets in your pantry or freezer that have any added sugars or sweeteners. For the next 2 weeks, they're not an option. Stash them with those carbon-belching snacks you purged if that's easier for you.

- Eliminate any drinks with added sugars or artificial sweeteners. Choose 100 percent fruit or vegetable juice instead of "punches," "drinks," "sodas," or "ades." Swap sugary coffee drinks for black coffee or green tea.

- Avoid noncalorie sweeteners and sugar substitutes (even natural ones) and foods that contain them. They are listed as ingredients such as sucralose or acesulfame potassium, along with newcomers such as erythritol, stevia, and agave nectar.

- Avoid alcohol for 2 weeks. After that, you can include (if you can afford the extra calories) up to one (5-ounce) glass a day of wine for women and up to two glasses for men for health benefits.

COOL HOT SPOT #4:
COOK YOUR FOOD, DON'T BUY IT

"If the United Nations were organized by industry," said Michael Oshman, founder of the Green Restaurant Association, which provides green certification for restaurants throughout the United States, "restaurants should be sitting side by side with other businesses negotiating the Kyoto Protocol."[21]

Here is another of the most basic overlaps between leaner and greener living: Cook more often for better health and carbon savings, especially if you have Energy Star–rated appliances. And in today's economic squeeze, it will save your food dollar as well.

Taking food on the go (dining out, drinking out, snacking on the run) is a critical hot spot because it's a prime area of adding a bunch of "middlemen" to your food. All of these steps, of course, require fossil fuels and cough more carbon into the atmosphere. It's also an eating style with a high ratio of packaging waste and food waste, as restaurants dish up larger portions to create "value," or wrap up each part of your meal-to-go with all the accoutrements, such as tiny packages of ketchup, salt packets, and straws. Eating on the run is also a prime way that Americans get too many of the wrong types of calories. So if you are serious about getting lean, healthy, and green, it is essential to dial back dashboard dining. Period.

LEAN BENEFITS

When it comes to food choices, Americans are choosing the "dashboard dining" route more than ever before, which ultimately means we have much less control of what's on our forks. In fact, while the 2008 downturn may have softened these stats just a bit, according to the USDA's Economic Research Service, half of every food dollar is spent on food we don't make ourselves.

If you're like most Americans, you probably woefully underestimate how many calories or how much salt or fat is in your "on the go" meal. I know. I've run hundreds of "guessing games" at corporations around New England, and I saw it time and again; employees regularly guessed much lower when it came to things such as the number of calories in that morning muffin and coffee drink, that fast-food meal, or even that salad.

A healthy weight starts with healthy foods in healthy portions. The easiest way to keep track of calories and maintain the right portion sizes is to make sure everything you eat comes from your own kitchen. Otherwise, it can be a fast and furious slide into overeating.

In fact, study after study has shown that when people eat out, they are more likely to consume too many calories and too much saturated fat, trans fat, and cholesterol.[22] Further, experts estimate that between 75 and 85 percent of our total sodium intake comes from the processed food and restaurant food we eat. Diners on the go are also likely to eat too few whole grains, fruits, and vegetables.

Think you're smarter than that? Think again. Oftentimes these studies were conducted using faculty and staff (read: educated people) at university settings during regular mealtimes—not, as you may be tempted to think, overeager slobs with no self-control who were simply offered a free meal so researchers could see what they did.

"We all think we're too smart to be tricked by packages, lighting, or plates," wrote Brian Wansink, one of the world's top researchers on food psychology. "We might acknowledge that others could be tricked, but not us. That is what makes mindless eating so dangerous."[23]

The mega-portions, dollar menus, and other incentive pricing are building more than just brand loyalty to a restaurant; they are also helping to build your backside. Put another way, portion sizes are linked to pants sizes.

To repeat: Dining out does not get you lean. It's unfortunate, but even those well-intended menus that list calories alongside lighter options have been cast into doubt; a recent investigation by a news station (sampling from eight cities) found that dishes aimed toward weight-conscious consumers at some leading national chains contained as much as twice the calories and eight times the saturated fat as the restaurants claimed in their published information.[24] Cook your food yourself and you'll stay in ultimate control, and consider eating out a splurge in every sense—for your wallet, your waistline, and the planet. Health professionals have been telling you this for years, but ditching the grab-and-go lifestyle also creates immediate savings in one of the hottest spots of our supersize American diet: our supersize waste.

GREEN BENEFITS

We've all seen it (and if we're really honest, we can admit we've all *sat* in it), that line at the drive-thru that creeps along, be it for a morning jolt of java at the local doughnut drive-thru or a dinner rush at a casual dining chain. And the line of SUVs, trucks, and cars spewing planet-warming exhaust in various amounts from their tailpipes, creeping along a drive-thru line and blasting AC or heat until their drivers can order some combo of artery-clogging, low-nutrition, high-carbon meals, represents perhaps one of the biggest dietary splurges on the planet.

The additional element of having all your food run through what is essentially another production system, and the river of materials, packaging, and petroleum that carries these convenience meals to you, pack on the carbon in much the same way that their oversize portions will pack on the pounds.

Restaurants are the retail world's largest energy user and, according to Pacific Gas and Electric's Food Service Technology Center, use almost five times as much energy per square foot than any other type of commercial building. Restaurants also produce far more garbage every day than almost any other retail business.[25] Although there are certainly some notable exceptions, as an industry, much remains to be done before it merits any sort of green bragging rights.

And then there is the matter of any leftovers that you throw away. Food waste, when it goes to a landfill, emits methane, a powerful warming gas that's 23 times as potent as carbon when it comes to warming the planet (of course, that's true for the home cook as well, which is something to consider, but having worked in restaurants for 14 years, I doubt most people are tossing out similar volumes of food at home).

Americans, despite having only 5 percent of the world's population, are the planet's worst trash offenders, contributing about 40 percent of the global garbage scene. All of this dashboard dining is creating supersize waste even by American standards. A disposable lunch creates between 4 and 8 ounces of garbage every day, which can add up to 100 pounds per person each year.[26] With establishments annually churning out an average of 50,000 pounds of waste, and using around 300,000 gallons of water every year, restaurants are one of America's largest waste-generating and water-hogging industries.

Eric Schlosser's groundbreaking book *Fast Food Nation* already got people thinking about the true cost Americans have to pay to subsidize that popular dollar menu, and now it's time to add the global warming piece on top of that. Bags for kids' meals, toys and wrappers, drinks, straws, and cardboard containers bring you what amounts to around a 5-minute, super-high-calorie eating experience, and then end up in a landfill, where they emit the powerful warming gas of methane.

As with sugar, I'm certainly not suggesting people abstain completely. Dining out can be pleasurable and delicious, and many restaurants around the country are leading the way toward healthy, sustainable foods that support healthier, more sustainable communities. But all things considered, restaurant food, especially fast food, is, as a category, seldom a green choice, so it's something to limit as much as possible. While there is now virtually an entire spectrum of "food on the run" these days, from fast-food joints to fine dining, from coffee bars to doughnut drive-thrus, for the next 2 weeks, focus on eating food from your own kitchen as much as you can. One of the fastest ways to get back to a healthier body and weight, and to a lower carbon lifestyle, is to use the kitchen more and the drive-thru less.

TAKE ACTION NOW

- Skip the dashboard dining for the next 2 weeks and head back to the kitchen instead. Take meals to work with you, pack lunches and snacks for your kids, and eat (or make and take) breakfast before you leave the house in the morning. To keep it easy, it may help to focus on a few big, one-pot meals with lots of leftovers. Chili, soups, pasta dishes, or slow-cooker meals can all make fast eating at home a snap. (You can get started with some of the menus starting on page 228.)
- Yes, you *can* get a tasty, healthy, more sustainable meal on the table in under 30 minutes. Many TV celeb chefs have

shown us how. Pick up a fresh cooking magazine or cook-book that can inspire you in the kitchen.

■ *A lighter shade of green:* If you absolutely have to dine on the run, avoid meat and cheese (choose vegetarian instead); drink water, herbal tea, or coffee; and make sure you don't toss a morsel of food. Ideally, choose a restaurant that is certified by the Green Restaurant Association (which ensures that the restaurant has key sustainable practices). There are more than 350 of them across the United States. Log on to http://dinegreen.com/restaurant_guide.asp to find out what's near you.

As famed personal coach Tony Robbins said, "Hope is not a strategy." Achieving the body and health that you want will require that you summon the discipline to make a few changes, but therein lies the good news: A few well-considered changes is all it takes.

While installing solar panels or rethinking the family wheels may not be in your immediate future, with food it's different. The fact is, sometime in the next couple of hours, you will have to eat. And you will have a choice to make. A choice that doesn't need to wait for car manufacturers, politicians, or nations to act. A choice that depends only on one person: you.

Now let's move on and consider what is the single most important aspect of your diet's carbon footprint: the type and amount of protein on your plate. Are you ready to jump in with me? Fantastic. Welcome to your new style of eating. It's time to become a flexitarian.

FOCUS ON THE FOOD CHAIN

Where you choose to eat on the food chain is one of the most important decisions you make when it comes to your health and your weight. It's also the single biggest area of your "food footprint," which is why we're tackling it straightaway.

Here in Part II, which covers week 3 of the diet, you'll discover how to enjoy a better ratio of healthful, leaner, sustainable proteins. It's a strategy that works on land (eat plants rather than animals) and sea (those smaller fish at the bottom of the food chain are actually lean *and* green). It even works in the air (avoid any protein that's flown to you in an airplane)!

Here's an overview of the specific action steps you'll be taking.

GET STARTED NOW: REAL, SIMPLE SOLUTIONS TO START LOSING TODAY

1 **TRIM THE AMOUNT OF ANIMAL PROTEIN IN YOUR DIET.** Enjoy smaller portions when you serve meat (e.g., serve 4 to 5 ounces of beef instead of 8 to 10 ounces), and heap on lots of great side dishes of veggies, beans, and salad. Serve animal proteins weekly or monthly instead of daily and add more plant protein in its place.

2 **MAKE SUSTAINABLE MEAT AND POULTRY CHOICES AT THE MEAT COUNTER.**

3 **GET THE DISH ON SUSTAINABLE FISH.** See page 91 for a list of action steps.

CHAPTER 4

BEEF

The Protein Problem:
Why This Nutrient Matters Most in Your Diet

66 Which is more responsible for global warming: your BMW or your Big Mac? Believe it or not, it's the burger. 99

—Bryan Walsh, *Time*

YOUR LEAN AND GREEN PRESCRIPTION
Beef: up to 6 ounces a month

INCLUDE

Sirloin, tenderloin, top round, or 90 or 95 percent lean ground beef

Greener: minimal packaging, all natural (no antibiotics or growth hormones), grass fed, local, and organic

AVOID

Kobe beef (An ultra-luxe splurge. Considered the "foie gras" of beef because of its rich marbling of fat; to earn the Kobe beef designation, it must be slaughtered in Japan.)

Beef from Brazil or other tropical areas where cooling rainforests are burned to make way for burgers

High-fat cuts (including brisket and ribs)

Ground beef less than 90 percent lean or fast-food burgers

Processed deli/lunchmeats

Worst offenders: highly processed meats, meats with a high degree of packaging, meat flown in an airplane to reach you, meat raised in another part of the world

---

Now before we begin, I have a confession to make. As a dietitian, I hesitate to launch this section of the book with advice to "eat less" of something. For many people, that's a cue to grab a voodoo doll of their dietitian and begin pricking away. After all, who wants to be told to eat less? Certainly none of my clients, and probably not you. Truth be told, if beef weren't such a hot button, I definitely would have been tempted to bury this chapter further back in the book. But it is. So take a deep breath and read on.

First, the basics. In my experience, most Americans seem to drastically overestimate how much protein they actually need. How much is enough? Most adults need just under 1 gram of protein for every kilogram of body weight, or about 4 grams of protein for every 10 pounds of body weight (for the average 150-pound man, about 60 grams). That translates to about 15 percent of total calorie intake, and it's worth pointing out that most Americans easily meet this requirement without even trying.

So you may be asking, If we're getting enough already, why the push to protein-rich plant foods? Remember that protein comes not by itself, but bundled in a package along with many other nutrients. And that package makes all the difference.

Trust me. The goal of this chapter is not to turn you vegetarian (although if you want to, that's fine, too). Rather, it is to welcome you to the world of the flexitarian, a critical key to leaner, greener living.

The term *flexitarian* was coined sometime in the '90s, but it's steadily finding its way into the mainstream. A "flexitarian" is someone who follows a primarily plant-based diet, with limited amounts of meat, fish, and chicken. Back in the day, your hippie cousin or younger sister may have called herself a "semi-vegetarian" or "almost vegetarian"; these essentially mean the same thing.

I like to use "flexitarian" because the idea is to keep it easy and flexible, for the inevitable bumps in the road that life will hand you. Clients like it because it doesn't sound as restrictive to them, which makes it more doable. I also like it because, after all, you aren't a vegetarian. You are a flexitarian, who can still have the occasional splurge of red meat—but you now recognize that it's truly a splurge in every sense.

LEAN BENEFITS

Eating lower on the food chain is a remarkably easy means to getting lean fast because, ounce per ounce, plant protein foods are significantly lower in fat and calories than animal protein foods. As a general rule of thumb, I suggest aiming for at least 60 percent of your protein to be coming from plant sources: This means incorporating more high-protein plant foods such as beans, legumes, tofu, and whole grains into your diet and thinking of animal proteins as weekly instead of daily additions.

And if you have wavered in your "staying power" in the past, take heed. Eating lower on the food chain may also be one of the best strategies to not only lose weight, but to *keep* it off. We'll delve more into the slimming benefits of those La Luscious Legumes in Chapter 7, but a 2007 study found that people following a diet free of animal products lost almost three times as much weight as those following a conventional low-fat diet, and they were able to maintain that advantage even 2 years later.[1] While this research looked at people who excluded all animal products (vegans), when you become a flexitarian, when you eat lower down on the food chain more often, you will get closer to reaping these types of weight benefits.

Remember that packing your plate with plant foods is an easy way to keep volume high while trimming calories. What's more, this type of eating pattern also improves your intake of disease-fighting phytonutrients and fiber (did you know that constipation is the number one gastrointestinal complaint to doctors in America?), as well as vitamins A, C, and E, selenium, and zinc.

So what's to gain besides an easier means to weight loss? Plenty. A growing body of research continues to pump up the notion that plant proteins are also healthier for your body than animal proteins. A few highlights: People who eat less animal protein tend to be thinner, and they have lower rates of heart disease and colon cancer. What's more, people who abstain from beef have lower blood pressure and cholesterol levels than those who eat it.[2] And a National Cancer Institute study found that when men were asked to add 1½ cups of beans a day to their diets, they lost 10 pounds in the first month.[3] Tastes great, and *more* filling.

Here's another immediate bonus: A flexitarian diet is also cheaper. (Remember college, when you loaded up on rice and beans because it was cheaper than meat?) In fact, globally speaking, a meat-heavy diet is a rich person's diet, and it's linked directly to what health experts call diseases of affluence: heart disease, obesity, type 2 diabetes, and high blood pressure.

But we're not the only rich ones anymore. As countries such as China become more affluent, they are clamoring for more meat in their diets, too. The question is: Heart health aside, what will the impact be as more countries demand to eat like Americans?

While I don't know how it will exactly shake out with China per se, chew on this: Can you guess how long it would take before the Costa Rican rainforest would be completely gone if it were cleared to produce enough beef for Costa Ricans to eat as much beef, per person, as the people of the United States? One year. What about Indonesia? Three and a half years.[4]

I have a 1-year-old and a 3-year-old. Framing our consumption in these terms stops me in my tracks. I can't help but shudder at the thought that if people around the world adopted an American eating style, what might the world look like for my kids? Who should be eating this way at all? Am I suddenly a socialist? No, I conclude. I'm just a mom who's beginning to realize just how much food choices matter.

Clearly, focusing on the food chain matters. Take a look at "Focus on the Food Chain to Save Money, Calories, and Carbon" below and you'll see three things. Number one, you can see how easy it is to

FOCUS ON THE FOOD CHAIN TO SAVE MONEY, CALORIES, AND CARBON[5]

PROTEIN SOURCE (4 OZ)	COST PER POUND	CALORIES	GRAMS OF PROTEIN
80 percent lean beef, cooked	$3.69	288	26
Porterhouse steak, broiled	$9.99	388	24.7
Firm tofu, raw	$2.26	94	10.1
Lentils, cooked	$1.00	115	9
Quinoa, cooked	$4.49	111	4
Chickpeas	$0.80	143	6

reach your daily protein goals (and how a person can blow through his or her total daily needs with one good-size piece of meat at dinner). Number two, you can see how easy it is to shed hundreds of carbon-heavy calories from your weekly choices by swapping to plant proteins. And number three, as promised, you've also now freed up a bunch of money for your new lean and green lifestyle. Switching to plant-based proteins not only saves fossil fuel energy, but it's also a means to cutting your grocery bill and one of the fundamental pillars to creating better health within yourself.

Flexitarian living is also a powerful way to keep your cardiovascular system healthy. Why does that matter? Heart disease is the leading killer in America, accounting for almost 40 percent of total deaths a year.[6] In fact, in the time it took you to read this chapter so far, one or two Americans have died from heart disease (about one every 34 seconds). And millions more are saddled with chronic heart disease that requires medications and lifestyle adjustments that eat away at their vitality and quality of life.

Of all the research that has examined the relationship between diet and health, one of the most consistent findings is that limiting red meat to a couple of times a month at most is the best strategy for optimal cardiovascular health.[7] Comprehensive, groundbreaking studies such as the best-selling *The China Study* discovered consistent evidence that all pointed to the same finding: *People who ate the most animal foods got the most chronic disease, and people who ate the most plant foods were the healthiest and more likely to avoid chronic disease.*[8] The research also points in the exact same direction when it comes to healthy aging, balanced energy, improved digestion, and reduced inflammation, one of the underlying mechanisms in many chronic diseases. My own personal experience has been the same; I've found that there's a tremendous sense of energy and vitality that people often gain as they begin to move to a more plant-based diet. And that's a wonderful plus, because "improved energy" is one of the things most people are looking for.

All of this, in short, is why so many of the leading health organizations recommend a diet based mostly on plants, with limited amounts of the *right* kinds of animal protein.

So rest assured, if you enjoy downing a good steak or burger once in a while, that is fine. In fact, if it's truly "once in a while," it's perfect, because it's now striking a much better balance and represents a more sustainable eating style on *all* fronts.

Now that you have a clear picture of the lean benefits, let's moooove on to looking at the eco-costs of our heifer habit.

GREEN BENEFITS

Let's get right to it: Bovines are right up there with smokestacks as critical to the global warming crisis (otherwise, like I said, I'd have tucked this chapter deep in the back of the book).

"Livestock are one of the most significant contributors to today's most serious environmental problems,"[9] according to a 2006 report by the United Nations. The report found that livestock account for 65 percent of human-produced nitrous oxide, a gas that has nearly 300 times the warming power of CO_2. In fact, beef consumption is *so* important to your personal carbon footprint, in addition to your own long-term health, that if you change only *one* thing about your diet, let it be this: Eat less beef. A lot less. Starting right now.

The United States is the number one beef producer in the world; in 2005 Americans downed an average of 67 pounds per capita per year. As I've said, this aspect of our diet is part of what gives Americans the largest carbon feet in the world. If you choose foods lower on the food chain, it's an instant way to go greener. "The Meat-Carbon Connnection" below helps put the exact carbon savings into context.

THE MEAT-CARBON CONNECTION[10]

HOW MUCH MEAT DO YOU EAT?	CUT BACK BY THIS	AND SAVE THIS
Well below average	2 oz/day	819 lbs CO_2/year
Below average	4 oz/day	1,637 lbs CO_2/year
Average	8 oz/day	3,274 lbs CO_2/year
Above average	16 oz/day	6,548 lbs CO_2/year

American meat eaters, on average, are responsible for a personal contribution of 1.5 more tons of carbon dioxide per person than vegetarians each year;[11] multiply that by the 290 million meat-eating Americans, and it's a larger carbon output than many countries.[12]

Okay, so by now you get it. Too much beef, bad. Plants, good. Now let's see how easy it is to move from knowledge into action without creating mutiny at the dinner table.

"Here we had been thinking about switching lightbulbs and walking to the bus stop as part of our New Year's resolution to live a greener lifestyle, and I had no idea that shopping for food could be such a big part of our impact," said Jennifer Waddell, a director with Timberland Corporation in New Hampshire. When her children were given homework from a "global warming" unit, the family decided that they would take steps to go greener. Among their many lifestyle changes, they've decided to skip their weekly steak-on-the-grill meals and have instead transformed their regular "make your own chili night" into a vegetarian feast, full of fun toppings the kids can pile on themselves. That's an instant carbon-cutter. Fifty-two fewer beef-centered meals a year multiplied by a family of five. Simple. Powerful.

So now let's get back to why that big burger is such a problem for global warming. According to researchers at the University of Stockholm, the average cheeseburger (including bun and the usual toppings) releases somewhere between ½ to 1 pound of carbon per burger, depending on various inputs (say, gas versus coal power, whether the cukes were grown in a greenhouse or not).[13]

While these figures are based on European metrics that don't equate exactly to the United States, if you consider that the average American eats about three burgers a week, and that there are 300 million of us doing so, that translates to 75,000 to 150,000 tons of carbon released into the atmosphere as a result of this collective burger habit. This estimate doesn't even include that "enteric formation" I was telling you about; add this into the equation, and the number climbs even higher.

Put another way, a 2008 study by the National Institute of Livestock and Grassland Science in Japan found that 2.2 pounds of beef (about eight quarter-pounders' worth) creates the same amount of carbon dioxide emitted by the average European car every 155 miles; that's enough energy to light a 100-watt bulb for nearly 20 days.[14]

I point out these facts not as a beef basher, but as your nutritionist. I understand that Americans love beef—truth be told, I love to eat beef from time to time. And I understand that a significant segment of America makes its living in the cattle industry. But I also understand that we are in an era of new realities and, like many sectors of our economy—automotive, energy, electronics—these new realities will require some industries to adapt to change. To me, this is an opportunity to insist on the highest quality of beef, to shower praise on beef companies with sustainable, ecofriendly practices, and to bring our consumption, at the very least, to levels that are compatible with the best health we can give ourselves and our children.

If you're a die-hard beef fan and are still having trouble imagining life with fewer burgers, remember this. No matter what your current eating habits, you can have immediate, significant savings by just cutting *back*. So often people lose the chance to be good because they don't think they can be great. I used to see this "black and white" thinking all the time when I was actively counseling clients in Boston.

WHY IS BEEF LIKE AN SUV?

It turns out that just about every step of conventional cattle production is warming to the planet. First, you have to grow their feed, which takes energy. It also takes pesticides and fertilizers, both of which are petroleum based. In addition, cattle need water (*lots* of water) and other agricultural "inputs" and management.

That's just the input side. Then there is what can delicately be referred to as enteric formation. This is known more commonly on the street as burps and farts. Then there is what can delicately be referred to as the waste issue. This is known more commonly on the street as poop. Believe it or not, cow burps, farts, and poop are a significant contributor to global warming.

Pound for pound, beef is an inefficient way to deliver calories as compared with plants. Consider the following:

IT TAKES: [15]

About 7 pounds of corn and 2,500 gallons of water to produce 1 pound of body weight on cattle

About 1,600 fossil fuel calories to produce 100 beef calories (compared to about 50 calories to make 100 plant calories, which is about 32 times more efficient)[16]

More than 200 gallons of fuel to raise a 1,200-pound steer on a feedlot[17]

About 5 times as much water to grow feed grains as it does to grow fruits and vegetables

GLOBAL IMPACT

33 million: the number of cars needed to produce the same level of global warming as is caused by the methane gas emitted by livestock and their manure in the United States[18]

Eating a low-meat diet uses 41 percent less energy and generates 37 percent less carbon than a typical diet.[19]

19 percent: the proportion of methane contributed by cows and other livestock (methane is 21 times more potent in global warming than carbon dioxide[20])

In 2000, livestock in the United States produced about 3 trillion pounds of manure, which is about 10 times as much as people produced.[21] Roughly half of all irrigation water in the United States goes toward livestock.

SAVE CARBON NOW

The Center for Science in the Public Interest (CSPI) has a fun and easy tool to calculate your impact of eating animal products (available at www.cspinet.org/EatingGreen/calculator.html). You type in how many typical servings of different animal products you eat each week, and it gives you a yearly calculation of your personal impact. If you are an average American eating 64 pounds of beef per year, your personal impact is the following:

- 2.3 acres of land needed for animal feed

- 42 pounds of fertilizer used to grow this feed

- More than 14,700 pounds of manure created by the animals you ate

- More than 282,000 gallons of water used[22]

If you cut out just 3.5 ounces of beef (about 1 serving) per week, you'll save more than 6 pounds of fertilizer and 1,500 pounds of manure.

So if you're having trouble letting go, consider this: A great goal is to just cut your current meat habits in *half;* that would have a major carbon and health savings. So if you currently eat beef six times a week, trim it down to three or four and know you've done something good. According to one study, the substitution of 1 pound of bread for 1 pound of beef monthly throughout a year by US citizens would save energy equal to that contained in more than 120 million barrels of oil.[23]

And as you will soon learn, there are greener types of beef—organic, grass-fed beef is a different story for both your health and your carbon count. So while Americans definitely need to eat less, the good news is you can now put some of those newly freed-up dollars into the highest-quality, cleanest beef you can afford.

Ultimately, what you eat is your choice. But it turns out that the consequences of those choices run deeper than most of us have previously thought. So now that you know, will you shut your eyes but continue to open your mouth? Before you answer, let's turn to two other major protein sources: chicken and pork.

CHAPTER 5

POULTRY, PORK, AND LAMB

66 As a professional athlete for 11 years, I never realized how changing what I put into my body would so dramatically affect how I would feel and perform. After eliminating junk food and switching to a primarily vegan diet, I have much better energy, improved recovery, and I feel better than ever! 99

—Tony Gonzalez, nine-time NFL Pro Bowl, All-Pro tight end

YOUR LEAN AND GREEN PRESCRIPTION
Poultry: 4 ounces, up to 3 times a week
Pork or Lamb: up to 5 ounces total, once a month

INCLUDE
Whole chicken and turkey (cooked with a small amount of clean fat, not deep fried)

Chicken and turkey breast or thighs (bone-in or boneless). (If you cook with the skin on, as I do to retain moisture, just be sure to remove skin before eating.)

Lean ground turkey or chicken breast (ask butcher to make sure there's no skin included, which increases fat and calories)

Naturally raised pork products that contain no added hormones or antibiotics in the following cuts: tenderloin, boiled ham, Canadian bacon

All-natural and/or organic turkey, chicken, or ham deli slices (get it sliced fresh to save on packaging; slice it extra thin so you can pile it on while staying slim)

All-natural lamb (leanest cuts include shank, loin, and shoulder) trimmed of all visible fat

Greener: minimal packaging, vegetarian fed, locally raised, and organic

LIMIT/AVOID
Highly processed products such as chicken nuggets, breaded or fried chicken products, chicken or turkey sausages, frozen chicken dinners (even all-natural or organic ones)

Breaded and stuffed with high-carbon ingredients such as cheese and ham

Traditional air-cured meats and sausages (I suggest "limit" as opposed to "avoid" with this one) that contain no nitrates, nitrites, or preservatives (examples include foods such as real prosciutto or air-cured salami)

All-natural bacon or sausage (can still be high in fat, sodium, and calories)

AVOID
Conventional bacon, sausages, cured ham, fatty cuts of pork such as spareribs, hot dogs, and fatty deli meats that contain pork (such as bologna)

In 2007, Tony Gonzalez captured the attention of the sporting world when he switched to a primarily plant-based diet, including small amounts of chicken and fish. Working with my good friend and colleague Mitzi Dulan, a dietitian who is the nutritionist for the Kansas City Chiefs and Kansas City Royals pro teams, Gonzalez began to follow a diet that challenged one of the oldest-held myths in the athletic world: Animal protein is necessary for peak performance.

That season Gonzalez went on to land a place in the NFL history books for most touchdowns and receptions of any tight end in history. Dulan's formula for success? One that's closely aligned with Go Green Get Lean Diet principles: "I encourage all athletes to incorporate more plant-based foods into their diets, aim to eliminate processed foods, and choose organic whenever possible," she says. "Not only is it better for their health and the environment, but as I have watched Tony Gonzalez dramatically change his diet to mostly vegan, I see how it can improve performance when done correctly." In fact, Gonzalez was so successful and so happy with the results that he and Dulan are penning their own book outlining the secrets of his success as a step-by-step guide for athletes. So much for the argument that being a flexitarian is fringe.

Of course, after you read about beef in Chapter 4, you may have thought, "Well now that I know about red meat, I'll just opt for more white meat like pork and chicken." Wrong. Despite what the pork industry wants you to think, *pork is red meat, folks.* But you'll see that I've grouped pork and chicken together in this chapter, along with lamb, because after my exhaustive hammering home of the problems with beef in the last chapter, I thought I'd give you a little break. Plus, none of these animals have the same carbon consequences to their burps and farts, so it's a bit more straightforward. Let's first consider where chicken, pork, and lamb fit into a lean and green lifestyle, and then we'll address one of the central questions of a greener lifestyle, the big "O." Organics.

The Word on the Bird

So let's talk turkey for a minute (and chicken, too). We're now jumping right to the "best" when it comes to a lean and green overlap at the meat case. According to 2004 USDA estimates, Americans consume an average of 60 pounds of poultry per capita (in contrast to 66 pounds of beef). Poultry's popularity is easy to understand; it offers a versatile, economical, easy-to-cook protein staple for many food traditions around the world. It's included on the vast majority of diets, whether they're for weight loss, heart health, diabetes management, or optimal health. And in my experience, it sometimes provides an easier transition for die-hard meat eaters to stomach than instantly turning to tofu. An added plus: It may be surprisingly easy to source something local to you.

LEAN BENEFITS

Why is poultry a better pick than red meat? Two primary reasons: less artery-clogging fat, and fewer calories. Also, there seems to be something about grilling, barbecuing, or frying red meat that increases the presence of potentially cancer-causing compounds (called heterocyclic amines), which researchers suspect may be another reason why red meat is connected to cancer risk.

Several major studies have found that eating fish and chicken (along with more fruits, veggies, beans, and whole grains) and lower amounts of beef and processed meats is linked with significantly lower rates of heart disease.[1] More than several, actually. Hundreds. It's an eating pattern that is emerging as one of the primary ways to ensure not just a longer life, but one that's also more likely to be free of the disease, disability, and medication that are mistakenly being accepted as a normal part of aging. And because this type of eating pattern is tasty and varied (and still includes some meat and fish), it won't, as my father once worried, be a Draconian eating plan that "just makes it *feel* like you're living longer."

Or perhaps you're already well versed in the latest nutrition science. If so, you'll know that many leading health organizations and their respective diet pyramids have been encouraging people to eat chicken instead of red meat for years. And the *Harvard Medical School Guide to Healthy Eating* includes eating fish, chicken, beans, and nuts for protein as one of its top dietary strategies for health and longevity. Turns out poultry is also cooler for the planet. Cool.

GREEN BENEFITS

When it comes to carbon footprint, after being vegetarian or vegan, eating poultry is the next coolest type of diet, about three times as energy efficient as beef and five times as efficient as pork.[2] As I've already said, much of this advantage comes from the lack of any backend (literally) warming gases, as well as fewer inputs needed (food, water, etc.) to create the bird on a per-pound basis. This is why it is the most liberally included of all the animal proteins on the Go Green Get Lean Diet. If you're going to be a true flexitarian, then try to eat even less, choosing more beans, legumes, and tofu instead.

These figures, from a 2006 University of Chicago study, show how much fossil fuel it takes to produce your protein. Note, however, that this is just the input side; it does not include the "output" warming gases methane and nitrous oxide associated with beef, which pack an additional 9.48 grams of CO_2 per calorie into beef's warming plume. When that's factored in, suddenly beef becomes much more carbon heavy than lamb and pork, and even the tuna and salmon.

This table also shows you why, even in the sea, where you eat on the food chain matters. Look, for a moment, at the fuel efficiency of

CHECKING THE FUEL GAUGE OF YOUR DINNER PLATE: HOW MANY FOOD CALORIES DO YOU GET FOR 100 FOSSIL FUEL CALORIES?[3]

FOOD	CALORIES	FOOD	CALORIES
Chicken	18.1	Lamb	1.2
Milk	20.6	Herring	110
Eggs	11.2	Tuna	5.8
Beef (grain fed)	6.4	Salmon (farmed)	5.7
Pork	3.7		

herring compared to salmon and tuna. Why the big difference? Food chain. Herring live close to the shore in large quantities (along with other small fish such as sardines, mackerel, and anchovies), so they're much more energy efficient to harvest when compared to, say, a tuna that's far out at sea. A greener catch, if you will. This is great news, because all these little buggers—herring, sardines, mackerel, and anchovies—are also super-rich sources of heart-healthy, anti-inflammatory, beautiful-for-the-skin omega-3 fats! Ready for some more lowdown? Because they are low down on the food chain, they are much less likely to be contaminated with mercury and PCBs than their salmon and tuna kingpins. And as an added feather in your eco-cap, their large populations mean no issues about dwindling populations (at least, not yet). How fabulous. But I'm getting ahead of myself; there's a lot more on that to come in the next chapter.

Of course, when I say that poultry is leaner and greener than red meat, I'm referring to poultry as a whole food—actual chicken breasts and thighs and stuff like that. In my opinion, organic, local, and free-range are the best choices if possible, but even if you buy the traditional chickens, that's okay. But I am *not* talking about highly processed products such as chicken "nuggets." Who knows what the actual carbon footprint is when you take chicken parts, process them, add a litany of other industrial ingredients, stamp them into various cartoon shapes, plunge them into a dizzying array of plastic wrapping that's then put in a cardboard box, and then plunge *that* into a freezer until it's shipped in a truck a couple hundred or a couple thousand miles to a freezer aisle near you? But hey, global warming is a big problem, what can *you* really do about it?

For starters, you can make the Ginger Chicken Kebabs on page 247 instead.

Pork: The Other Red Meat

I have to hand it to the marketing team at the Pork Board; they have done an incredible job of convincing America that pork is just another white meat. But pork is actually classified as a red meat by the USDA. While this may be more than you ever wanted to know, the

WHAT DOES THE FOSSIL FUEL DENSITY OF FOOD REALLY MEAN?

In the nutrition world, two metrics are used to evaluate the nutrition status of a particular food.

Energy density of food: how many calories you are getting in relation to the amount of food you eat

Nutrient density of food: a measure of the nutritional value of the food as compared to its calories

These two concepts help you quickly determine whether a food is a good trade-off for calories and nutrition involved. For instance, a 12-ounce can of soda has a high energy density (150 calories) but a low nutrient density (basically all high-fructose corn syrup, or possibly refined sugars)—not exactly a winning combination for losing weight and boosting health. In contrast, a 10-ounce bag of spinach packs loads of vitamin K, beta-carotene, lutein, iron, and fiber into each bite, all for 65 calories. In other words, it has a high nutrient density but a low energy density, which is why it is listed on practically every healthy eating plan you have ever seen.

But there is one more metric that needs to be added as we see the deep connection between our food choices and the global warming crisis: the fossil fuel density of food. What was the fossil fuel cost of bringing that food to your plate? How does this relate to the calories versus the nutrition? Is it drenched in petroleum, like that pineapple fruit basket you just express shipped from Hawaii as a thank you to your personal assistant, or is it tinged with a much smaller amount of gasoline because you live on the coast and walked out to the public beach early this morning and caught something yourself?

Something to start thinking about.

---

classification of red meat versus white meat has to do with how much myoglobin (a protein that helps bring oxygen into the muscle) is present. Pork is classified a "red" meat because it contains more myoglobin than chicken or fish. When cooked, it does become lighter in color, hence the appealing idea of calling it "the other white meat," especially given the immense boost to pork's image as a health food.

Pork is "livestock" along with veal, lamb, and beef, and livestock are considered "red meat." So it's really best to eat only limited amounts of this stuff—about once or twice a month tops, if you want to get healthy. Less if you really want to be a flexitarian.

LEAN BENEFITS

Because of the fact that pork is red meat, it is especially important that you stick to the leanest cuts when you do indulge. As a general guide, anything with the word *loin* in the title is a good indicator that it's a healthier choice that will keep calories in your target range. Ribs? Bacon? Sausage? While it may feel like hog heaven to indulge, if you eat these kinds of foods on any sort of a regular basis (as they are usually loaded with artery-clogging fat, sodium, and preservatives), make room in your day planner down the road for some serious stent work.

When it comes to pork products, be sure to choose all-natural pork without sodium nitrite or sodium nitrate; these preservatives are often used to keep pork's pink color looking fresh, as well as to inhibit the growth of harmful bacteria. Hot dogs, lunchmeats, sausages, and bacon are just a few of the places where these are commonly added. But there's a catch; both of these ingredients have been linked to cancer. A recent University of Hawaii study, for instance, found a 67 percent higher risk of pancreatic cancer in subjects who consumed the most processed meats,[4] and other studies have found links with higher rates of stomach and colon cancer.[5]

Think it will be too pricey to go "au natural"? Think again; it's easier than ever to find all-natural alternatives nowadays. (One of my personal faves is Organic Valley; they make amazing bacon and sausages. You may be able to find something delicious and fresh that's more local to you as well.)

Another way to steer clear of nitrites and nitrates, and to ensure you're getting the highest quality of pork possible, is to seek out traditional meats made using clean, low-tech, time-honored methods such as salt and air curing to deter bacterial overgrowth instead of nitrites and nitrates. Many of the traditional pork products from Europe, for instance, are made this way, but increasingly there are more and more traditional handcrafted pork products showing up on this side of the Atlantic as well (in fact, famed chef Mario Batali's father, Armandino Batali, owns an amazing shop in Seattle that specializes in this stuff, appropriately named "Salumi Artisan Cured Meats"). However, even these cleaner versions should still be savored in modest portions only on occasion (and if so, include them toward your monthly Prescription), as they can still be high in salt and saturated fat.

So whether the economy is flush or tanking, cut back a bit. Insist on high-quality pork products, and get more bang for your buck by relishing the taste. You can use some of your freed-up food dollars (remember, you're eating less fast food, less sugary stuff, and less beef) to invest in a couple of higher-quality, amazingly better-tasting items that are better for you and the planet.

GREEN BENEFITS

The triumvirate of beef, pork, and lamb is included sparingly on the Go Green Get Lean Diet because of the health drawbacks we've already mentioned as well as the higher carbon count. All three of these meats independently have a higher carbon footprint to produce as compared to poultry or eggs, and are hands down a hotter choice than anything from the plant kingdom. Just remember this: A diet including red meat was found to be significantly more fossil fuel dense than one that included only poultry.[6]

Lamb: A Higher-Carbon Splurge

Now, if you're like most Americans, you probably don't consume all that much lamb. According to the USDA, in 2005 Americans consumed less than 1 pound per person a year. However, it is a mainstay in many delicious (and healthy) cuisines around the world, so if you come from another tradition (i.e., Greek, Turkish, or Indian), or if you simply enjoy foods from these countries, you may eat more.

LEAN BENEFITS

As with all red meats, look in your butcher's case for the leanest cuts and trim all visible fat before you eat. One plus that lamb has going for it is that it is usually grass fed, so the meat is likely to have a healthier ratio of omega-3s to omega-6s than grain-fed animals. As you'll see in Chapter 8 when we delve into "greener pastures," animals that eat grasses and clovers tend to have higher levels of anti-inflammatory omega-3 fats in their meat than do those fattened on a feedlot or in a factory farm. This has important benefits to your own health, which we'll discuss a bit later. In addition, growth hormones are not traditionally used on lamb, which limits your exposure to them even if you buy conventional cuts. (While human studies have yet to show specific health outcomes from consuming meats containing added hormones or antibiotics, as a mom, I prefer to be conservative and eschew them as much as possible.) And as many of these are relatively recent additions to our food supply, as a nutritionist and foodie, my personal belief is that "less is more" when it comes to what's in your food.

GREEN BENEFITS

Lamb, as you saw from "Checking the Fuel Gauge of Your Dinner Plate" on page 68, is the least energy efficient of all the red meats to produce. But if you are like most Americans, lamb is a much smaller component of your diet than beef, poultry, or pork, which means it's going to be a much smaller part of your personal carbon footprint than foods that you include daily. And many cuisines enjoy small amounts of lamb alongside large amounts of plant food, as opposed to the "steak on a plate" approach Americans seem to prefer.

If you do eat lamb, be sure to eat it in place of your pork or beef guideline, not as an addition. Otherwise, that flexitarian lifestyle is going to increasingly resemble that of a solid meat eater.

But what about the "local" issue? Does it matter as much if you don't eat it regularly anyway? Experts have been wrangling about the answer for years. The short answer is that the jury is still out.

In 2006 a study from New Zealand found that it was actually four times more efficient for a Londoner to buy lamb raised in New

Zealand as opposed to Britain. The study (no doubt in response to Europe's interest in "food miles" labeling, as 50 percent of New Zealand's exports are in food and beverages) credited all those advantages of climate and geography of New Zealand for saving an estimated 2,161 kilograms of CO_2 per ton of lamb.

Sounds like a closed case, right? Not so fast. While the study was "the shot heard round the foodie world," and journalists gleefully seized on the research as a counterpoint to all localism trends (and while it no doubt raised some good questions), the differences might not be explained solely by abundant rain falling softly on New Zealand clover fields. Firstly, the researchers didn't include estimates of in-country transportation on either side—from farm to boat in New Zealand and from boat to consumer in Britain. This would likely chip away at some of the savings. Secondly, much of the "energy advantage" New Zealand provides comes from the fact that Britain still derives much of its power from coal while New Zealand uses a high percentage of hydroelectric energy; these advantages are likely to decrease or vanish altogether in the future as Britain, like everyone else, tries to move to more renewable energy.[7] Thirdly, it's hard to overlook the fact that the study was conducted by people connected to agricultural interests.

To me, what this study does show is how complicated and contentious the issue of "green food" may well become in the years ahead. For now, it seems best to consider it with a grain of salt. For in all of my research and interviews conducted for this book with some of the country's (and the world's) top experts in green eating, one consistent theme I heard was this: Even if it's not *always* a hands-down winner, eating close to home is still one of the key approaches consumers can use to tread more lightly with food choices.

"The number of miles between Chile and the Carolinas will never change," wrote Helene York, director of the Bon Appétit Management Company's Low Carbon Diet Initiative, to me in an e-mail, "but on-farm practices and off-farm delivery systems can always get better. We have to invest in the future of great local food now."

The Big "O": Is Organic Better?

Let's turn, for a moment, to the issue of organics. You've already seen it mentioned several times, so before we move on, I want to provide you with a basic primer. I say "basic" because, to be frank, the big "O" is such a vast topic that it could easily be a book unto itself. Or at the very least, a chapter. Still, I'm going to try to give you "the basics" in a slightly shorter version; if you want more, I highly suggest Marion Nestle's *What to Eat* as one of the best books to make you an expert for the next time you step into the supermarket.

Organic is one of the biggest buzzwords in the food world these days. But the term covers issues as varied as the food supply itself: Is organic milk safer? Are organic strawberries better for you? And what about things such as organic french fries or organic cocoa-covered breakfast cereal? In fact, I recently received a call to be interviewed for a national fitness magazine about "the myth of organics." Unfortunately, "organics" was simply lumped into one big pile, and in my professional experience, there's a bit more nuance than that.

As a consumer, you have to ask whether organic is worth the extra money. Let's face it, organic sticker shock can hit the most dedicated of shoppers, especially in an economic squeeze. Is it better for you? And if you have a limited budget for organics, where should you put it?

Here are the key reasons why the Go Green Get Lean Diet emphasizes organic meats and animal products (always), and organic produce (if you can find it, to the extent you can afford), leaving the rest up to your own choice, economic situation, and value judgment. First, let's consider the lean side of the equation.

LEAN BENEFITS

While there's no research to date on whether organic products help you lose weight more than conventional ones do, what people often really want to know when they talk to me about organic food is

ORGANIC AT A GLANCE

Is organic safer for you? Organic products reduce your exposure to certain toxins, pesticides, and hormones in all food categories. In my opinion, that is a plus, especially when it comes to animal products. While all have been approved by the FDA, it is a personal choice and value judgment that is up to you (but worth noting: many of these are banned in Europe and other parts of the world).

Are organic foods healthier? For animal products, grass fed versus feedlot will likely be a bigger determinant of a product's nutrient profile. For fruits and vegetables, some research has found that organic produce does have significantly higher concentrations of certain phytonutrients and vitamins than conventional (but whether or not these translate into specific health advantages has not been proven). For the aforementioned cocoa-covered breakfast cereal and french fries, organic products may reduce your exposure to pesticides or toxins, but junk food is still junk food, even if it's all natural.

Is organic the greenest choice? Up until the farm gate, yes. But for both organic and conventional foods, packaging, storage, and transportation can add pounds of carbon and may also degrade nutrient value.

Will organic help you lose more weight? Not likely. Unless, perhaps, if the higher prices compel you to eat less.

whether it is more nutritious. I'm often asked, "Will I be healthier if I eat organic?" In a nutshell, probably yes. But in reality, the answer isn't quite so easy. But here are the reasons why I favor organics as the best choice for meat, poultry, and dairy products, as well as most produce.

Let's start by talking about organic animal products (meat, poultry, eggs, dairy, etc.). The primary reason organic, in my opinion, is better for you is because of what's *not* in it. Organic products do not contain added hormones or antibiotics, and all feed is vegetarian and certified organic. It's a personal choice, to be sure, but I believe we simply don't have enough definitive long-term evidence about the effects of ingesting conventional agriculture's "by-products," especially as it relates to children.

If we are what we eat, it's safe to say that animals are what they eat, too. And when it comes to cows, their milk and cheese and yogurt reflects the quality of their own diets. As I'll explain more fully in Chapter 8, cows that eat living grass and clover (their natural diet) incorporate greater levels of many different nutrients into their meat, milk, and cheese; several studies have found significantly higher levels of antioxidants, vitamins, and minerals in organic grass-fed animals than in conventional ones.

Grass-fed animals also are likely to have significantly higher levels of omega-3, which is a heart-healthy, anti-inflammatory fat. Studies have consistently found that grass-fed beef tends to be leaner overall and has from three to five times the heart-healthy omega-3 fats of its conventional counterparts.

I will go into more detail about this in Chapter 8, when we take a close look at the health benefits of conventional versus organic dairy products, but the vibrancy of the food of animals grazing the way they're supposed to on clean grasses instead of fattened up on corn is significant, and in my opinion provides a nutritional advantage.

Further, USDA-certified organic labeling requires that animals are traced from birth to slaughter (something many other countries and the European Union already do). This may give the consumer an additional margin of safety and assurance, because if there are any problems, your exact animal can be traced right back to the source. Organic animals might also reduce the risk of food-borne illness from contaminated meat, as the animals are raised under less-crowded conditions. Lastly, as cloned meat and milk products may be getting set to hit store shelves in the near future, choosing organic provides a clear means to avoid those if you have any doubts.

When it comes to the merits of organic fruits and veggies, first let me be clear about a few things. It's much better to eat conventional produce than no produce at all. As you'll see in Chapter 9 (which probably won't be earth-shattering news to you), there's overwhelming evidence that there are major health benefits to eating lots and lots of fruits and vegetables. Period. So that is your first step to leaner living (also greener living, as they're lower down on the food chain).

The second thing to be clear on is this: Soil quality and the amount of time it takes your food to get from "farm to plate" are far more important factors in determining nutritional value than an organic sticker. Food is only as rich as the soil it's grown in, and as time passes from harvest, certain vitamins (such as vitamin C and folate) and phytochemicals will begin to degrade, which helps answer one of the new quandaries of a global food system: "Which is better, a local conventional strawberry or an organic strawberry from China?" When I've asked chefs, the answer is always local. When I've asked moms with young kids, it wavers a bit more toward organic because they're concerned about pesticides and health. Like I said, eating involves trade-offs. But from a sheer nutritional value standpoint, that fresh local strawberry is likely to have retained more vibrant nourishment. Which is "best" is up to you.

Just for the purpose of comparison, let's imagine a scenario where we have the best of both worlds and all things are equal. Let's say you had your pick of organic or conventional, and both came from right next door to you. Is there a benefit to organic? The research seems to suggest there might be. A 2003 study in the *Journal of Agriculture and Food Chemistry* found that organic berries and corn contained 58 percent more polyphenols (the same wonderful compounds that give wine some of its health benefits) and more than 50 percent higher levels of vitamin C than did conventional.[8] Another study from the University of California, Davis, found that organic tomatoes contained greater than 80 percent higher levels of certain antioxidants and vitamins than did conventional.[9] And early results from the most expensive studies conducted on this topic (the Quality Low Input Food Project, a £12 million study funded by the EU involving 33 centers across Europe) are showing that organic fruit and vegetables contain up to 40 percent more antioxidants than nonorganic varieties, that organic milk contains more than 60 percent more antioxidants and healthy fatty acids, and that organic food contains higher amounts of minerals such as iron and zinc.

While researchers have yet to translate this difference into a specific health advantage (i.e., whether or not people who eat organic fruits and vegetables have lower rates of cancer than those who eat the regular stuff), it nonetheless adds one more plus to the possible health advantages of organic.

Then there's one last important benefit: Organic produce reduces your risk of exposure to pesticides and fertilizer residues.

GREEN BENEFITS

The largest "green" benefit of choosing organic is the immediate carbon savings that come with skipping all of the fossil fuel needed to manufacture, ship, and apply nitrogen-based fertilizers and pesticides. In fact, the creation of these synthetic fertilizers and pesticides used in conventional farming accounts for almost 40 percent of the energy used in all of US agriculture.[10] Because of the absence of such products, organic agriculture has carbon dioxide emissions that have been estimated to be 30 to 60 percent lower than conventional systems.[11] By way of example, consider that from June 2001 to June 2002, the United States used more than 12 million tons of nitrogen fertilizer, which is the energy content of 96.2 million barrels of oil.[12] Organic production doesn't use these.

Similarly, organic farmers rely less on machinery and more on labor-intensive practices to weed and harvest their fields. To study the impact, a 22-year study from the Rodale Institute determined that conventional farming methods require 3.7 barrels of oil per hectare of crop production, while organic farming methods used only 2.5 barrels of oil to produce the same crop yield. An added plus? Organic fields acted like a "carbon sink," storing at least twice, and up to three times, as much carbon as fields farmed using conventional methods.[13] Perhaps that's why corn and soybean organic farming systems produced 30 to 50 percent higher yields during drought years than did conventional.[14] Of course, many of these advantages disappear if those organic items are then put on a chilled airplane and flown 3,000 miles so we can nibble strawberries by a crackling fire in the dead of winter, but we'll get to that issue later.

What about cows? I've read lots of blogs where skeptics charge that grass-fed and organic production will require more land, and hence would be less efficient than claimed. Or that these cows take longer to raise, so they will be higher in carbon.

Here's why they're wrong: The science has shown that animals raised on good organic pasture are actually much *more* efficient to feed than animals raised on grain. A 2006 report by Cornell University's Organic Center concluded that organic grass-fed beef systems required 50 percent less fossil fuel energy than conventional grain-fed beef systems.[15] And while it does take them a bit longer to grow (10 to 20 percent longer to reach ideal weight), and they produce more waste during this time (about 60 pounds of manure per day), they still require less overall fossil fuel input.[16]

Organic grass-fed beef may carry a lower carbon footprint for another reason as well; those cows might just emit less methane and other "backend" gases when raised on more digestible grasses instead of grains. A Swedish study in 2003 found that organic beef raised on grass rather than concentrated feed emits 40 percent less greenhouse gases and consumes 85 percent less energy.[17]

While critics charge that organic farming has less productivity and therefore can't really feed our population, research has shown that the difference is actually very small; in fact, organic farms are nearly as productive as conventional. Plus, they leave the soil and water in much better shape.[18] What could be better?

Phew. I admit, all those numbers and stats can be daunting. After all, you signed up (presumably) to lose weight, not to become the next member of the UN's global taskforce, right? If you've read this far, great job. So let's leave the numbers for a while and start talking solutions.

First of all, before you start panicking that this is a diet for the elite and you can't afford organic so this must not be for you, let's dig a bit deeper into the way we spend our food dollars.

When the cost of food goes up, the American response is to trade down to cheaper brands. Underlying this automatic practice is a disquieting assumption about food's relative importance, or unimportance, in our lives.

"Instead of practicing the peasant's art of turning humble fare into a nice spread, we merely substitute poor-quality ingredients," wrote Oregon-based chef Kelly Myers recently.[19] "This is a half-baked effort to eat the way we always have, but for less money."

If you ask me, Kelly Myers is spot-on with her take of the American food approach. Why is it that we immediately want to know how to cut corners on what we feed our children and our own bodies? As it turns out, there is a whole host of other "costs" that come with that decision. So here are some steps you can take right now to get you moving in a healthier and slimmer direction, all without blowing your budget.

TAKE ACTION NOW

- Be strategic in your purchases. You *don't* need to buy everything organic. If you're on a limited budget, the most important things to buy organic, in my opinion, are foods that come from animals, namely meat and dairy products. So start there. (Here's another tip I use to save money: A certain supermarket in my area sells organic meats, but because it's the most expensive market overall in town, I go only once in a while to stock my freezer with meat. It's worth the cost, but I know I can find a better deal on other pantry items somewhere else.)

- Focus on the "dirtiest" produce. No, I'm not talking about potatoes that still need a good scrubbing. By "dirty" produce, I'm referring to the Environmental Working Group's published list of the fruits and vegetables that typically have the highest levels of pesticides on them. To the extent you can afford, this should be the next place you put your dollars. Log onto their Web site and download the guide at www.foodnews.org/walletguide.php. They also have a list of produce that contains the *lowest* amounts of pesticide residues, which is where you can feel better about buying conventional. Just be sure to wash and peel it before eating.

- Start sourcing locally. Log on to www.eatwild.com, which lists more than 800 US and Canadian farms raising pasture-fed eggs, meat, and milk. Check out www.localharvest.org to locate a CSA or farmers' market near you.

- Stick to the season. Buying local and seasonal will help keep your costs down and the nutrition high.

- Bargain shop. Once the domain of high-end markets such as Whole Foods, organics have hit the mainstream. You can now find organics from Albertsons to Walmart, to the discount clubs such as BJ's, Costco, and Sam's Club—at a price that's less likely to give you sticker shock.

- Cash in your other savings. Remind yourself of the other places where you have freed up food dollars. You're using the kitchen more and the drive-thru less (ka-ching!), you've laid off the sweets (ka-ching!), and you're now a flexitarian (ka-ching!). Remember, now that you're eating less meat *overall,* you can buy more expensive meat, just less often.

- Continue the shift to lighter living. Add the following to your next shopping list: canned beans (such as chickpeas, black beans, and cannellini beans), dried beans and lentils, all-natural chicken stock (for cooking up those yummy beans), extra-firm tofu, and frozen edamame beans.

Ready to move on with me? Great. In the next chapter, you'll learn whether or not you should try to wrangle your own dinner. Let's move on to the Fish and Game Department.

CHAPTER 6

FISH AND GAME

Is Catching Your Own Dinner Better for You and the Planet?

❝People can still savor things like wild salmon and ahi tuna, but they need to begin seeing them for what they really are: a splurge, a luxury item, rather than casual daily fare.❞

—Corey Peet, aquaculture research manager, Monterey Bay Aquarium

YOUR LEAN AND GREEN PRESCRIPTION
6 ounces protein per day
Fish/seafood: up to 4 ounces, up to 2 times per week*
Game and fowl: up to 2 times per week (in place of chicken, pork, or beef)

INCLUDE

Herring, sardines, anchovies, mackerel, and US-farmed catfish, barramundi, and tilapia

Fish and seafood whose populations are abundant, well managed, or farmed in sustainable and environmentally sound ways, such as frozen wild Alaskan salmon; striped bass; and US farmed shrimp, clams, oysters, and mussels

Any game and fowl that is not endangered, is local to you, and is hunted legally with all necessary permits, such as elk, deer, pheasant, rabbit, duck, and partridge (or even moose, if you're in Alaska!)

Grass-fed buffalo (But look closely: Only about 2 percent of commercially sold buffalo or bison is grass fed; 98 percent is fattened on feedlots with grain, and in this case the health advantage vanishes.)

Greenest: Something you or a friend caught yourself

LIMIT

Fish flown overnight to get to your plate (e.g., fresh wild Alaskan salmon, certain sushi). Ask your restaurant or fishmonger how the fish arrived.

Any fish listed as an "alternative" on a sustainable seafood list for your region

Highly processed game products (e.g., commercial sausage or jerky), or game that is naturally raised but shipped overnight to you directly from the source

AVOID

Breaded and fried fish items (e.g., "fish sticks," fish fillets, fish 'n chips)

Any fish listed under "avoid" on a sustainable seafood list for your region

Exotic meats ("bush meat"), any illegally hunted game

*Except for children under age 15 and women of childbearing age (thinking of becoming pregnant, pregnant, or nursing)

Wouldn't it be cool if I told you that whatever you can catch, shoot, or trap yourself can become a delicious and healthy part of a lean and green lifestyle? That you'd burn tons of extra calories before dinner as an added plus? Doesn't it seem to make intuitive sense that "living off the land" is leaner and greener?

Believe me, I wish it were that simple. The reason this chapter lists your specific fish recommendations right at the top is to try to keep it as simple for you as possible. But that's the catch—there's nothing really simple about your catch. As with organics, there can be a dizzying amount of nuance if you start digging. So for the purposes of this book, I am going to keep it reduced to the basic information you should know to get started.

Fish and Seafood

While it's relatively easy for a health expert to pan the steak in the name of cleaning up your diet, with fish it's more complicated. No other food source so perfectly frames the greater debate—weighing the environmental cost of a food against the nutritional benefits it offers—as does fish. That's because fish and seafood (along with bottled water) is one area where "lean" and "green" don't neatly overlap.

For years I, like many of my health-professional colleagues, have been enthusiastically recommending regular fish intake, even putting wild salmon up on a pedestal of perfect eating. But it's becoming clear that when it comes to green, there's nothing sustainable about the idea of every American downing fresh wild Alaskan salmon twice a week. According to the Worldwatch Institute, the fishing industry harvested about 141 million tons of seafood globally in 2005, which was *eight times as much* as in 1950. Ask any expert in the fish or aquaculture industry if they think these levels are sustainable, and you will get one answer: no.

We need to rethink our fish and seafood choices, and quickly.

LEAN BENEFITS

Here's the dish on fish: Without a doubt, fish and seafood are super healthy for you. Ounce for ounce, fish and seafood tend to be lower in calories than most meat and poultry options (see the table below). They also have more omega-3 fat and little or no saturated fat, and tend to be a rich source of important minerals such as selenium, magnesium, and zinc. Many of the world's healthiest diets contain regular amounts of fish and seafood, and it is a key strategy in the fight against heart disease.

You can see how these swaps will help whittle your waistline quickly without sacrificing taste. Eat more than 3 ounces and the savings are even bigger.

Particularly, it is the omega-3 fatty acids found in fish that are so healthy, especially eicosapentaenoic acid (EPA) and docosahexaenoic acid (DHA). These essential fatty acids help reduce blood clot formation, lower the risk of stroke and heart attack, fight inflammation (an underlying component of many diseases), and are critical in healthy brain and eye development.[1] In short, these fats are a key ballast in our diets for optimal health, and fish (especially fatty fish) are one of nature's richest sources of them.

That about sums it up from the pure nutrition side. Chances are, unless you've been living in a cave somewhere for the past decade, you've already heard that you should be eating fish twice a week to significantly cut your risk of heart disease. But here's the first catch. Unfortunately, because fish swim in waters that we use as drains and septic systems, there's a dirty underbelly to eating fish; the biggest concerns involve PCBs or methylmercury contaminants. As tiny

SLIM DOWN WITH THESE SUSTAINABLE SWAPS[2]

CHOOSE THIS (3 OZ)	INSTEAD OF THAT (3 OZ)	AND SAVE THIS
Wild Alaskan salmon, 160 calories	Beef loin, broiled, 280 calories	120 calories
Grilled shrimp skewer, 84 calories	Grilled meat kebab (using sirloin), 207 calories	123 calories
Wild striped bass, 105 calories	Breaded chicken cutlet, 252 calories	147 calories
Farm-raised US catfish, 129 calories	Spareribs, 279 calories	150 calories

fish are gobbled up by bigger and bigger fish (that whole "food chain" thing again), these toxins increase in concentration, which increases concern about possible dangers to people who eat them. If you are eating sport fish, it is critical that you check your local and state advisories.

Large carnivorous fish (which are essentially the lions of the sea) such as swordfish, shark, tuna, and salmon are prized around the globe, but because of where they sit on the food chain, these species have also been shown to be the most susceptible to contamination.[3] In response to this fact, our government cautions vulnerable populations, such as children and pregnant women, against eating these large and predatory fish regularly, if at all.

So what's a consumer to do? Looking *just* at the contamination concern for a minute (we'll get into green later), as a dietitian, my opinion is that for most people, the health benefits of eating fish far outweigh the possible contamination risks, and that's for nearly everyone *except* women who are of childbearing age (pregnant, may become pregnant, or nursing). According to a joint recommendation by the EPA and FDA, eating fish up to two times a week can be part of a healthy diet. In other words, keep your risk in perspective; if you're an adult, your risk of dying from heart disease is much greater than your risk of having toxic complications from moderate fish consumption. Remember what I said in Chapter 4: Heart disease is the leading killer in America by a large margin. And for what it's worth, according to the EPA, how you handle your fish matters when it comes to contaminants. You can actually cut your cancer risk in half by scoring the salmon fillets, grilling or broiling them, letting the juices drip away, and then removing the skin.[4]

GREEN BENEFITS

As you focus on your food chain in week 3, you no doubt are already beginning to see how the same rules apply when it comes to seafood. So when in doubt, use the food chain to guide you at the fish counter; it's an easy rule of thumb that will land you squarely in the leanest and greenest overlap of what to eat. When I attended the 2008 Monterey Bay Aquarium Sustainable Seafood Institute, the nation's top aquaculture and sustainability experts (my "fish peeps," as I call them) were recommending everyone eat fish lower on the food chain (such as anchovies, herring, sardines, and mackerel). This strategy is another of your ultimate "lean and green" overlaps, as they're easier to fish (greener), much more abundant (greener), and healthier, because while their lower rank on the food chain means less toxins, they still offer those heart-healthy omega-3 fats like fish higher up on the chain (such as salmon and tuna). An added bonus? They'll save you even more green at the checkout.

Now let's move from concerns about the quality of the fish and consider the impact those fish have on the environment. Let me start by saying that whether you choose farmed or wild fish, each choice has trade-offs, and unfortunately there is no "perfect" solution. When it comes to fish farming, a key strategy is to *choose plant-eating rather than meat-eating fish*. Herbivores such as catfish, tilapia, and barramundi that are farm raised, while lower in omega-3s than salmon, provide a leaner and greener alternative to any of the red meats we just covered. US-farmed clams, mussels, and oysters land squarely on the greener plate as well.

Where carnivorous fish are concerned, it's logical that one of the biggest issues is that of feeding; it takes from 2 to 10 pounds of wild fish feed to produce just 1 pound of farmed salmon. At a ratio of between 2:1 and 10:1, you can see why so much energy is required just to produce their "salmon chow."

Tuna farming is even worse. Because 15 to 25 pounds of wild fish are required to produce just 1 pound of farmed tuna, tuna farming may just sit right up there with Kobe beef production in terms of questionable practices. Farmed fish also require an intense water management system, and all that fish poop needs to be dealt with as well. Finally, all of these fish need to be kept in a narrow window of constant temperature through growth, transport, and storage until they are delivered to the consumer.

Of course, on a global scale, fish farming standards vary wildly depending on the country and the degree of government oversight. There are some truly visionary people working in aquaculture in the

United States today (I met several of them in Monterey) who are devoted to finding sustainable ways to produce commercial fish. This is a good thing, because the stark reality is that we will have to rely on aquaculture as part of the solution.

So is wild greener? Certainly, many of the inputs such as water, food, and temperature are taken care of compliments of Mother Nature, which is a plus. But how green the catch is varies from species to species. For wild fish, there are the energy costs associated with heading out to sea and catching the fish, processing it, packing in ice, and then transporting that fish fresh around the world to various locales (restaurants, markets, wholesale, etc.). Depending on the fish, this may well be by airplane so it can show up on menus from coast to coast in a matter of hours.

It's not a surprise that a 2006 University of Chicago study found that the most energy-efficient fish to eat were small fish that live in large numbers close to shore eating plants rather than other fish (examples include herring and sardines). Other similar research has extended "low-carbon" status to other seafood, including mussels and clams.[5] As I said before, these small fry are also some of the safest to eat in terms of mercury and PCBs. This provides a bright spot on the horizon for consumers; if some fish are a high-carbon, energy-intense luxury food, the good news is that there are many other options that make for a more sustainable dish. Eating a variety of different types of fish and seafood is also a sound strategy to minimize your risk of PCBs, mercury, and other contamination.

You may have noticed in the last chapter that I didn't mention fish at all in the organics debate. This is because organic doesn't really mean anything when it comes to fish. Of course if something is dangling at the end of your fishing pole and you are standing by the ocean, you might rightly assume that fish is "organic" in the traditional sense, but it still might be contaminated with toxins.

But what about farmed fish? you may ask. "Organic seafood and fish farming currently has no standards set by the USDA," explains Dane Klinger of the Blue Ocean Institute in East Norwich, New York. For a variety of reasons, seafood was left off of the table when the USDA was finalizing its organic standards, so any seafood labeled organic is based on that seller's (or an independently run certification company's) own definition. This means that someone in another country could raise fish according to their own definition of organic and ship it to the United States for sale under that label.

That's why right now, even though there are clear pros and cons between wild and farmed fish, your safest bet, in my opinion, is to "go native" when it comes to freshwater fish and shellfish by choosing US-farmed products. Alternately, if you shop at a very high-end supermarket with a strong sustainability focus, chances are that the fish counter has already done the work of scouting out the best global sources. But by choosing native, you can take comfort in the fact that the United States has a much more stringent set of regulations in place than many parts of the world (such as China).

Shrimp is a case in point, as it's one of the "big three" in terms of American consumption (along with tuna and salmon). Next time you're at the fish counter or freezer aisle, check the zip code on that shrimp. Or more likely, you'll see a country of origin; most of the shrimp these days is coming from Asia, where mangrove swamps are being destroyed to feed our appetite for shrimp. Think you're far removed from the impact on the mangrove swamps? Let me ask you, have you ever been to Vegas? If so, have you ever eaten from one of their ridiculously cheap buffets? If so, have you ever proclaimed

WHAT ABOUT FRESHWATER FISH?

Common sense, of course, would suggest that a good old "back to the land" approach—heading to your local waterway and catching something your-self—would be best for a lean and green diet. But after a visit lasting several hours to the EPA fisheries advisory Web site, clicking on state after state to see if this approach would work, one thing became abundantly clear: Unless you live in Alaska or Wyoming, most of us shouldn't be fishing in freshwater as part of a lean and green strategy. The issues around contamination, mercury, and PCBs run down to literally nearly every last fresh waterway in America. Idaho's advisory suggests that if you catch fish from certain lakes, you should bring that fish to a laboratory (which they list) and pay a fee to have it tested for mercury before you eat it. As if.

Nineteen states have virtually all their waterways under advisories. In state after state, I clicked on one town after another, and all of them came up telling me it was unsafe to feed virtually any fish to my young children, and that at most I (as an adult not planning to have any more children) could have only several ounces once a month. Even if I fished around the various streams and reservoirs in the outlying areas of my home in Park City, Utah (a rural region that many people might consider "remote"), these warnings blazed back at me from the EPA Web site. As someone who grew up in an avid fishing family in Massachusetts, where we still enjoy striped bass, lobster, and bluefish from the Atlantic Ocean during the summer, it was saddening and shocking. And while ocean fishing (for now, at least) is still possible for many species, it still requires that you become informed about the particular fish in your area. Bottom line? Catch and release is the best way to enjoy freshwater fishing.

"what a bargain!" as you piled your plate high with shrimp before heading back to the slots? If so, consider this: Las Vegas alone consumes a whopping 60,000 pounds of shrimp per day.[6] I can't help but wonder what the carbon footprint might be of *that*.

Nothing is wrong with indulging in fun foods, sometimes in ridiculously fun amounts, from time to time. But in America, we've completely lost sight of what is "moderate," even on a daily basis. We demand huge portions of food for bargain prices, and it has deeper implications than just spoiling the shrimpfest in Vegas.

But let's get back to salmon, that magical fish every dietitian has been raving about for years. Overall, wild salmon is a greener bet than farmed. In fact, wild Alaskan fisheries earn high marks for sustainability from even the most stringent environmental groups, so the leanest and greenest overlap here is to choose wild salmon that's been frozen or canned at sea. Further, several studies have found that farmed salmon, because they are carnivorous fish, are higher in PCBs and other industrial chemicals than wild.[7]

What types of carbon savings are we talking about? Salmon that is fresh and airfreighted has about 10 times the carbon impact of salmon frozen at sea.

TAKE ACTION NOW

- Get the facts, but focus on the fish you like to eat. It's not necessary to memorize the details of a 10-page-long national seafood guide. Most of us stick to the same couple of fish, such as salmon, shrimp, and tuna. Learn the greenest choices within the types of fish you eat the most.
- Get the dish on (sustainable) fish.

    Text it. Take advantage of the Blue Ocean Institute FishPhone: Whether you're seated in a restaurant or standing at the fish counter in a market, send a text to 30644 with the message *FISH* in all caps, followed by the name of the fish you want to know about. The Blue Ocean Institute, one of the leading pioneers of sustainable fish, will tell you immediately if that fish is eco-friendly or not.

    Become a card carrier. Download a pocket seafood guide that's specific to your region from Monterey Bay Aquarium's Seafood Watch Pocket Guide (www.mbayaq. org). Alternately, find your fave fish on Blue Ocean Institute's Seafood Guide at www.blueocean.org or on the Pocket Seafood Selector at www.oceansalive.org.

IF YOU DON'T EAT FISH:
OTHER WAYS TO GET YOUR OMEGA-3S

Perhaps you're part of the group most susceptible to the health risks posed by potentially contaminated fish, or you're just wary of consuming fish two times a week. If you want to sidestep the issue of fish altogether, there are other ways to get healthy omega-3s (particularly DHA and EPA).

Fish oil supplements. For maximum heart benefits, look for a supplement that provides 1,000 milligrams each day of omega-3s in the form of EPA and DHA. Choose supplements that contain the largest amount of EPA and DHA per capsule. Read the label; you may need to take two in order to reach this amount. (For example, a 1,000-milligram capsule may contain 250 milligrams of EPA and 250 milligrams of DHA, which adds up to 500 milligrams, or 0.5 gram, of omega-3 fat, so you would need to take two.)

Note: Be sure to check with your physician before starting any new supplement, especially if you have existing heart disease or are currently taking any medication.

Foods rich in alpha-linolenic acid. Alpha-linolenic acid (ALA) is converted in our bodies to EPA and DHA. Although they aren't converted as efficiently as fish, foods high in ALA still certainly add benefit. High-ALA foods include spinach, walnuts, soybeans, canola oil, flax meal, and flaxseed oil.

Fortified eggs. There are a handful of eggs on the market where hens are fed flaxseed or fish oil to boost the amount of omega-3 in the egg. Look for eggs that contain at least 50 milligrams of DHA apiece, such as Eggland's Best eggs. Gold Circle Farms eggs have 150 milligrams each. While this is only a small amount, the eggs can be part of an overall strategy.

- Find a reputable source. While Country of Origin Labeling (COOL) is set to go into effect in October 2008, it's still a good idea to get to know your fishmonger, and ask questions. A 2005 *New York Times* investigative piece found that only one out of eight types of salmon being sold as "wild" (and at a premium price) actually fits the bill.[8]

- Stop the market demand for unsustainable fish. Let your favorite restaurant and supermarket and fishmonger know you won't be purchasing any fish on the "avoid" list of your seafood guide.

For most people, the real benefit of swapping beef for fish is that it realigns their fat and calorie intake to be much healthier; you are cutting calories, decreasing saturated fat, and sometimes increasing omega-3s in one fell swoop. But it's important to note that you can *also* do this by becoming a flexitarian. By eating lower on the food chain, you'll also be cutting calories and saturated fat; you don't solely have to rely on eating fish twice a week, every week, as some magic bullet. A greener diet means enjoying smaller amounts of sustainable fish.

Wild Game and Fowl

Whereas fish has a litany of other concerns, with wild game it's pretty straightforward. Because game is fed by Mother Nature and not Big Oil, it sidesteps (for now) the sustainability and contamination issues that come up with formal animal production operations. It may not be a stretch to say that, if it is part of your cultural or culinary heritage, wild game can be a lean and green superfood. In fact, if you do hunt, it can be an inexpensive and healthy way to include meat in your diet. If wild game isn't part of your heritage, that is absolutely okay, too, but if you do have a chance to benefit from some of what Mother Nature has to offer, it makes lean and green sense for a variety of reasons.

LEAN BENEFITS

Stepping aside from the ethical issues of hunting (which are beyond the scope of this book, and I respectfully leave the reader to his or her own opinion), the health benefits of game for the body and the planet are superior to those of red meat produced conventionally. Animals are what they eat. Wild game is leaner and has a healthier fat profile than conventional livestock because it moves more, it's not fed a weight-gain diet, and its food sources often are organic grasses and foliage, so its meat has less artery-clogging fat and more antioxidants. Meat from grass-fed animals can also contain two to four times the amount of heart-healthy omega-3s that the meat of feedlot animals contains, in addition to providing the same amounts of iron, zinc, and many B vitamins as conventional meat.[9] Further, leaner meat tends to have fewer calories, making it easier to stick within your caloric budget. And perhaps just as important is what's *not* in the meat; because the game is raised by Mother Nature, it's free of administered growth hormones, antibiotics, and other additives that we just talked about in the last chapter when we considered the health benefits of organic.

THE SLIMMING POWER OF GRASS-FED GAME[10]

PRODUCT (3 OUNCES)	GRAMS OF FAT	CALORIES
Grass-fed bison (buffalo), sirloin	4.8	145
Venison, tenderloin	2	127
Beef, sirloin, select	7.5	175
Pork, loin, boneless	8.2	182
Chicken, skinless, thigh	9.3	178
Lamb, sirloin, boneless	9.1	183

Because it's not part of our conventional food system, game is an extremely low-carbon addition to your diet. While there may still be some petroleum involved in, say, driving out to hunt and storing it until you're ready to eat it, the fact remains that your protein source was fattened by Mother Nature instead of a factory farm feedlot, so much less oil was involved in the transaction. When done the right way, it also means you're helping to maintain a healthy ecosystem.

GREEN BENEFITS

If you are open to it and have access to game, it can be a healthy addition to a lean and green lifestyle, especially if it is local to you and part of your heritage (as it is for me, growing up in a hunting family, where all I wanted was a normal Purdue chicken like everyone else on our street, rather than some pheasant my dad brought home and my mom tried to pass off as chicken). Living in Utah, we have elk in our freezer right now (compliments of my dad) for delicious tenderloin—amazing in winter with a cherry sauce using dried Utah cherries—and ground elk meat that we use for burgers, chili, and a Bolognese meat sauce over polenta in wintertime. Do I also go to the local supermarket and purchase regular meat on occasion? Of course. But I do it less often.

If this sounds completely foreign to you but you are interested in dipping your toes in, game eating is becoming a bigger trend in restaurants as well—many chefs have made wild game more mainstream for Americans through cookbooks and cooking shows, and many restaurants across the country now offer locally sourced wild game, with venison consumption doubling nationwide in the past 4 years. If, on the other hand, this sounds completely primitive or otherwise unappealing to you, just stick to your standard Prescriptions and move on to the next chapter.

As an aside, please note that the Go Green Get Lean Diet considers game to be something that is hunted locally, in accordance with all permits and laws. This does *not* include exotic meats or animals from other countries, especially any endangered animals. Such meat is just plain mean.

So if hunting your own game isn't for you, what about all of those online and mail-order wild meats? Rather than scooping up plain old beef at the supermarket, is it better for the planet (and your health) to express ship gourmet venison sausages or grass-fed beef from across the country in a container, chilled, overnight to your door?

Here's where things get murky, and the truth is no one really knows, as there is not yet an exact carbon calculation on that one. But here is my suggestion: If it's in your supermarket sitting next to your beef or pork, see where and how it was raised. The closer to grass fed and organic, the better.

If you're ordering it online, the carbon footprint may be higher. While from a health standpoint it's preferable to eat grass-fed, organic animals (no matter how you get it), relying on meat or wild game from far-flung locales is not a recommended long-term strategy for greener living. Buying these from a catalog or Web site increases packaging, cooling, and food miles logged. And doing this as a long-term strategy seems to violate the spirit of treading more lightly on the planet, having less, and using less. See if you can find meat of a comparable quality that's raised more locally.

But if you don't see it in your market, ask for it. Supermarkets want to carry what they know will sell. The Wild Idea Buffalo Company in South Dakota, for example, is doing amazing work at restoring the native Grass Plains by using buffalo to naturally reestablish this ecosystem. Their product is a lean and green superfood—healthy grass-fed bison with Mother Nature doing the work of raising them. Right now they only sell their meat directly to the consumer, but they would love to sell it in supermarkets as a more sustainable strategy. "Consumers simply need to learn that most of the buffalo meat right now in the supermarkets is conventionally raised, so in fact their meat looks a lot more like feedlot cattle in terms of saturated fat and calories," says Dan O'Brien, one of the company's founders (www.wildideabuffalo.com).

Congratulations. If you've read this far and have been implementing the "Take Action" steps along the way, you have already done a tremendous job in resetting your path toward a healthier, slimmer, greener life. Fantastic. If you're like most of my clients, you are probably already experiencing higher energy levels, may have reduced constipation (as you've added more plant foods), and have seen the scale shift in your favor. Now, let's consider some of the leanest and greenest protein sources of all, the foods you will be adding more of to your new lifestyle: beans, legumes, and nuts.

WHY LEAN PLATES ARE GREEN PLATES

Can we eat our way to a greener lifestyle? Can we eat our way to better health and a better weight?

The answer is a resounding yes. *If* we make better choices, and *if* we consume a more appropriate amount of food and "food energy" from the planet.

Welcome to Part III of your program. Here in week 4, you will take the next important step of greening your plate. And you'll learn why lean plates are also green when it comes to beans and nuts, dairy products, eggs, fruits, and vegetables. While each chapter delves into great detail, here are the highlights, along with the specific action steps you can take *now* to start shedding pounds from your life.

GET STARTED NOW: REAL, SIMPLE SOLUTIONS TO START LOSING TODAY

1 **LOVE THOSE LA LUSCIOUS LEGUMES.** Eat more plant-based proteins, such as beans, legumes, and tofu, for the ultimate lean and green overlap.

2 **SEEK GREENER PASTURES.** Switch to sustainable dairy products, in more sustainable portion sizes. Reduce your intake of high-calorie, high-fat, high-carbon dairy products to lighten your loads even further.

3 **EAT LIKE A LOCAVORE.** Local and seasonal produce isn't a silver bullet for a global warming diet, but it does help cool your diet in many respects, and it has tons of nutrition and health benefits to boot. Eat "like a local" more often by loading up on local produce that's in season.

CHAPTER 7

THE LOWDOWN ON LEGUMES AND NUTS

❝I love the Go Green Get Lean Diet! Kate's plan has it all; it's super easy, it's tasty, it's fresh, it's easy to follow, and best of all . . . it works. And I love that it can work wonders for the planet, too.**❞**

—Summer Sanders, Olympic gold medalist, TV personality, and mom of two

YOUR LEAN AND GREEN PRESCRIPTION
6 ounces protein per day
Beans, legumes, and tofu: at least 1 cup per day (½ cup = 1 ounce protein)
Nuts, all natural nut butters, and seeds: 1 to 2 ounces per day

INCLUDE
Lentils—canned or dried (e.g., red, green, French)

Split peas and black-eyed peas—canned or dried

Beans—canned or dried (e.g., black, garbanzo, cannellini, navy, kidney, pinto, flageolet, lima, fava, soy or edamame, fat-free refried)

Tofu (calcium fortified) and tempeh

Greenest: Minimal packaging (i.e., dried or in bulk) and organic

All nuts, especially walnuts, almonds, pistachios, peanuts, cashews, pecans, and soy nuts. Enjoy them raw, naked, or roasted. (Minimally salted is okay if you don't have elevated blood pressure.)

All-natural nut butters: 2 level tablespoons is slightly more than 1 ounce (enjoy peanut, cashew, almond, and hazelnut)

Pumpkin, sunflower, and flax seeds

Greenest: Minimal packaging, more local to you, sustainably harvested, fair trade, Rainforest Alliance Approved or organic

LIMIT
Highly processed soy or bean products (e.g., frozen veggie burgers, soy "nuggets," soy cheese), because they are energy intense to produce

Nuts coated in sugary, flavored, or salty crusts (can boost calories and sodium)

Highly packaged nuts (e.g., single serving)

AVOID
Nuts not harvested sustainably. Nuts grown outside of the United States that don't have a Fair Trade, Organic, or Sustainably Harvested label.

The UN has spoken: Eating less meat may be one of the most effective ways to fight global warming.

How great, because going vegetarian (or at least flexitarian) is also one of the most effective ways to fight fat, heart disease, high blood pressure, and certain cancers. Remember, you don't have to swear off meat or your faves forever (besides, who really can or wants to do that?), but you can eat them less often, and in more responsible portions. That's the secret to not only getting the body you want, but also to immediately start taking a bite out of your carbon footprint. But if you've read this far, of course you already know all that. So I'll just briefly explain why beans and legumes kick butt. And help make your butt look great, too.

Those La Luscious Legumes

Legumes qualify as a lean and green superfood on many levels. In fact, beans are part of the "beautylicious" diet I give clients (along with those omega-3 fats) because their high fiber helps keep you regular and fights the belly bloat that comes with constipation. Plus, beans fill you up on fewer calories. So my advice is relatively simple—let beans be your no-brainer and enjoy at least 1 cup a day.

LEAN BENEFITS

Let's start with the research, which is clear. Vegetarians and vegans are the leanest people around the globe. While obesity rates are skyrocketing in the general population (two out of three Americans are overweight; one in three is obese), the obesity rate among vegetarians is much lower, ranging from 0 to 6 percent. To boot, vegetarians boast an average body weight 3 to 20 percent *lower* than that of meat eaters.[1] In fact, I had a client several years ago who dropped more than 150 pounds by switching from plates of chicken wings to plates of salad. He knew he liked VOLUME—he made that quite clear to me during his first visit—and was leery of me taking that volume away. So the trick was to give him volume while still managing calories. Produce was the secret. And it can be for you, too.

One particular research effort, the Oxford Vegetarian Study, compared 6,000 vegetarians to 5,000 nonvegetarians and found the vegetarians enjoyed healthier hearts as well as reduced risk of diabetes and a 28 percent lower death rate than the meat eaters. This study also found that the meat-eating men were twice as likely to be overweight and the meat-eating women 1.5 times as likely to be overweight than the vegetarians.[2]

Beans are also beneficial because they have a low glycemic index, which means they help keep your blood sugar stable longer. Why does that matter? When your blood sugar dips, it can trigger a hunger response. Eating more foods with a low glycemic index (and fewer with a higher glycemic index) can help keep your body's blood sugar/insulin response more stable. Not only is this better for your pancreas (which has to pump out a lot of extra insulin every time you toss back a food or drink with a high-glycemic load), but it's better for your backside, too. When you're trying to slim down, who needs to be at the mercy of a surprise hunger attack?

What's more, 1 cup of beans helps you meet a good chunk of both your fiber and your folate needs for the day. That's great news for women thinking of getting pregnant or anyone who's struggled with constipation or is trying to keep their homocysteine levels in check. Homocysteine is an amino acid associated with inflammation (high

WHY BEANS GET YOU LEAN

BEAN TYPE	CALORIES (1 CUP COOKED)	PROTEIN (GRAMS)	FIBER (GRAMS)	FOLATE (MICROGRAMS)*	GLYCEMIC INDEX
Chickpeas, canned	269	15	8	282	42
Kidney, canned	225	15	13	229	52
Lentils, dry	231	18	10	358	25
Pinto beans, canned	235	11	11	294	39

*The US RDA for adults for folate is 400 micrograms per day
(more if you are pregnant or lactating).

FOUR LEAN MEANS TO EAT BEANS

Looking for some easy ways to get lean with beans? Even if you're not a cook, beans are simple to include in your menu. Consider the following:

Nosh on hummus. See page 241 for a hummus recipe that offers a high-protein, low-calorie snack that's perfect with warmed whole wheat pitas or veggies.

Head south of the border for breakfast. Serve one scrambled egg with ½ cup black beans, a few tablespoons of salsa, and ⅛ of an avocado for a satisfying breakfast in 2 minutes flat.

Savor soup more often. Make your own concoction by adding some pureed beans or lentils to your favorite soup; it will give it a creamy texture and rich taste without the fat.

Supplement your sides. Mix lentils or chickpeas into side dishes such as rice or couscous to provide a hefty dose of protein and fiber.

---

levels are associated with an increased risk of heart disease, stroke, and peripheral vascular disease). Folate is one of the key nutrients that helps convert homocysteine into (benign) methionine.

Because there is no fiber in animal foods, as you begin to shift to a plant-based diet, you may find that your GI tract needs a few days to adjust. If so, that's perfectly normal; you can gradually increase your intake of beans and legumes each day until you meet your Prescription goals. Most people find that when they're eating the right amount of plant food, they're able to toss out their fiber powders and potions.

GREEN BENEFITS

The new green cuisine is rich in legumes for a reason; plant protein requires about $\frac{1}{10}$ the fossil fuel to produce, emitting about $\frac{1}{10}$ the carbon into the atmosphere.[3] In fact, they're so inherently green, here's my advice: When shopping, don't worry about finding the absolute greenest beans and legumes available. Focus your efforts where you'll reap much bigger carbon and calorie savings—in eating at a friendlier spot on the food chain, and fewer processed foods.

As you saw in Chapter 4, plant proteins are a much cheaper (and greener) source of protein when compared to meat, so whatever kind you choose is good. Soy, for example, is about 200 times more energy efficient to produce than beef. In fact, if just 20 percent of households in the United States and Canada swapped 4 ounces of soy for 4 ounces of beef each week, the water savings over a year would be enough to provide 10 gallons of drinking water to every single person in the world.[4]

So consider beans a no-brainer and move on. Spend your time and energy focusing on *other* areas of your diet where organic choices can have a bigger impact. Some other pluses of beans? They have a super-long storage life, whether canned or dried, so they're easy to always have on hand. Their meaty texture can be as hearty as beef, whether in soups, stews, burritos, or chili.

The single largest barrier to eating beans that I have seen in 10 years of working with companies and clients is this: Most Americans just don't really know what to do with them because they haven't been part of our meat-'n-potatoes heritage.

Nuts and Seeds

One of the biggest mistakes that I commonly see people make is to avoid eating nuts because they have mistakenly lumped them into the "fattening foods" category. In fact, the opposite is true.

Nuts are one of my best secret weapons as a dietitian; they're a food where indulgence and health deliciously overlap. They are nutrient powerhouses that are portable and last a relatively long time. High in protein, monounsaturated fats, fiber, potassium, vitamin E, and many trace minerals, they provide a winning combo of heart-healthy fats and proteins that can help curb cravings and keep blood sugar and energy levels stable for hours.

LEAN BENEFITS

When it comes to losing weight with nuts and seeds, the key word here is *modest* portions. Nuts contain a surprising amount of fat, so they rank somewhat high on the calorie scale (1 ounce of almonds, about 23 nuts, weighs in at 160 calories). Stick to one serving a day. A good rule of thumb is to think "airplane portions"; those little bags contain about 1 ounce.

Several studies have found that when nuts are regularly included in an eating plan, people are more satisfied and are able to stick with a healthier eating style longer.[5] The tastier the food, the easier it is to include it long term in an eating plan.

In terms of the other benefits nuts provide, several of the largest cohort studies, including the Physicians' Health Study, the Iowa Women's Heath Study, and the Nurses' Health Study, have shown that eating nuts several times a week significantly cuts the risk of heart disease and diabetes.[6] Other studies have shown that a daily dose of nuts significantly lowers "bad" LDL cholesterol. For all of my clients with high cholesterol I recommend including 1 ounce of nuts a day as part of a cardio-protective diet.

While all nuts can be part of a healthy diet, there are a few that stand out as superstars. Walnuts, for example, are the richest source of heart-healthy omega-3 essential fatty acids, which, as I've said before, have been found to protect the heart, promote better cognitive function, and provide anti-inflammatory benefits. Walnuts are loaded with powerful polyphenols and antioxidants that help fight disease, including the antioxidant compound known as ellagic acid, which research suggests helps fight cancer and support the immune system. And a study in the April 2004 issue of *Circulation* found that when walnuts were substituted for about one-third of the calories supplied by olives and other monounsaturated fats, total cholesterol and LDL (bad) cholesterol were reduced, and the elasticity of the arteries increased by 64 percent.[7]

Almonds are another nutrient powerhouse. They're rich in magnesium, potassium, manganese, copper, vitamin E, selenium, and calcium. In fact, ¼ cup of almonds has almost as much calcium as ¼ cup of milk. Plus, almonds are one of the best nuts for maintaining healthy cholesterol levels, as 70 percent of the fat they contain is the healthy monounsaturated kind.

Pistachios in their shells are another personal fave I suggest to clients. Thought to be one of the oldest cultivated nuts on earth (they are mentioned in the Bible, along with almonds), "pistachio" is the Italian version of the word *pistah,* which is Persian for nut. (Pistachios were imported from Italy as snacks after World War II.)[8] Pistachios pack some of the highest fiber of any nut (1 ounce provides 12 percent of your Daily Value), provide a hefty dose of lutein and beta-carotene, and are one of the richest nut sources of phytosterols, compounds that have been shown to help lower the absorption of cholesterol from other foods.[9] They can be roasted in their shells, and I love that; it means that they take a bit more time to eat, making that 1 ounce go a lot further (about 50 whole pistachios). They, too, have a super-healthy fat profile and are an excellent source of copper, manganese, and phosphorus.

All-natural nut butters are another winner in this category because they're not only delicious, but they go a long way toward helping you feel full and satisfied. Two level tablespoons is just over 1 ounce of protein. Plus, by sticking to all-natural, you avoid any trans fats, added sugars, and other unnecessary ingredients. On the other hand, avoid low-fat peanut butter; it often contains more sugar than regular peanut butter, so the *calories* are about the same, which means no weight-loss benefit (and you've swapped heart-healthy fats for sugar!).

Fortunately, all-natural peanut butter is super-easy to find these days. Almond butter is also a great swap (but it can be more expensive), and nowadays wonderful all-natural cashew and hazelnut butters are also becoming easier to find. But don't forget, portions matter! Two tablespoons of peanut or cashew butter weigh in at about 190 calories, and 2 tablespoons of almond butter at 200 calories. So don't use any more than this, tops. A little dab'll do ya.

GREEN BENEFITS

The nuts at your supermarket may literally be grown all over the world. Cashews from Mozambique or Nigeria, almonds from California, pine nuts from Italy, and Brazil nuts from South America are more common than ever. Because some nuts are grown in tropical

FIVE LEAN WAYS TO INDULGE IN NUTS

Nuts are one of the few foods where it's easy to find a delicious and easy way to include them at virtually any meal or snack. Here are some examples of five different ways you could meet your daily 1-ounce requirement.

■ Breakfast sundae: Add 1 ounce almonds to 1 cup fat-free plain yogurt and ½ cup fresh fruit.

■ Midmorning snack attack: Spread 2 tablespoons all-natural hazelnut butter on 5 whole grain crackers, or if it's fall, local apple wedges.

■ Lunch bunch: Sprinkle 1 ounce cashews on your tofu stir-fry or in your salad for crunch, staying power, and nutrition.

■ Afternoon delight: Savor 1 ounce walnuts with 10 dark chocolate chips.

■ Dinner rush: Enjoy pan-seared pistachio-crusted tilapia with grilled local seasonal veggies.

regions or developing areas of the world, they share many of the same sustainability issues as foods such as coffee, tea, and chocolate. So it's important that if you do buy nuts from another country, you buy sustainably harvested nuts if you want them to be green. We'll delve into more detail about sustainable splurges in Chapter 14. But in the meantime, when it comes to nuts, here are a few general rules of thumb to use.

■ Consider buying nuts grown in the United States. Pistachios, walnuts, and almonds are all grown in California. Pecans have a robust following in the South and Midwest, where they are grown. Macadamia nuts are grown in Hawaii. In addition, these choices mean that you're trimming food miles and not cutting down rainforest.

■ Shop eco-labels. Look for a seal certifying Fair Trade, Sustainably Harvested, or Rainforest Alliance Approved when buying nuts from overseas. These labels help you choose products that preserve those critical "carbon coolers" on the planet—tropical forests—rather than destroying them (more on this in Chapter 14). Cashews and brazil nuts are two examples.

■ Pare down the packaging. Buy nuts in bulk when possible (store them in your freezer to maximize shelf life) or choose products with minimal or recyclable packaging.

■ Go organic, especially when buying imported food. All things being equal, organic nuts have less fossil fuel density because of less input of fertilizers and pesticides. If you can afford them and have options available to you, they may make for a greener pick.

TAKE ACTION NOW

■ Get inspired with some fresh recipes for free! Log on to www.leanandgreendiet.com and print out some of the recipes with beans and legumes that tap into your culinary diva. Or head to www.wholefoodsmarket.com/recipes and explore Whole Foods' vast reserve of luscious vegetarian ideas (type "bean" in the search box and you will discover dozens of new ideas).

■ Load up on raw or naked almonds, walnuts, and pistachios. (I like to choose pistachios with the shells on to help keep portions in check.) Stash them in your freezer to keep them super fresh and lasting a long time.

■ Switch to all-natural peanut butter if you haven't already. Add another nut butter (such as almond or cashew) to the mix if you want a little more variety.

■ Find a 1-ounce container that you can tote around for your daily dose of nuts; stash it in your purse, glove compartment, gym bag, or office drawer. (An empty mint tin may be perfect.)

CHAPTER 8

DAIRY AND EGGS: WHY GREENER PASTURES MATTER

> "If you are drinking milk that isn't organic or doesn't have words such as 'no rBST' or 'hormone free' on the label, then you are drinking something that has been banned in Europe, Canada, and Japan."
>
> —*The Daily Green*

YOUR LEAN AND GREEN PRESCRIPTION

1 egg, up to 5 or 6 per week (1 egg = 1 ounce protein)

1 serving sustainable dairy product or dairy alternative daily

Up to 5 ounces cheese per month

Avoid all of the "creams": heavy cream and half-and-half, ice cream, sour cream, cream cheese. Think of these as high-calorie, high-carbon splurges to be enjoyed a few times a year, tops.

SERVING SIZE:

1 cup fat-free or 1% milk, soymilk, or rice milk (fortified with calcium and vitamin D)

6 ounces low-fat or nonfat yogurt, or soy yogurt (fortified with calcium and vitamin D)

1 cup nonfat organic cottage cheese

Greener: Milk and dairy products that are rBGH free, preferably local, and/or organic. Choose traditionally made, raw-milk, grass-fed cheese for maximum CLAs, antioxidants, and omega-3s. Also seek out products with minimal packaging (i.e., reduce your use of single-serving sizes).

Eggs that are organic, certified humane raised, and local (fortified with omega-3 if possible)

Greenest: A vegan diet with no animal products whatsoever.

Let me say up front that dairy, like fish, is a bit complicated. (Eggs are much more straightforward, so much of this chapter is dedicated to dairy choices.) Before we get into the politics of dairy, the somewhat confusing science, and the issues about organic and grass fed, let's start by keeping it simple. Here are the three primary reasons behind your Lean and Green Prescription as far as dairy is concerned.

Reason #1: Focusing on the right amounts of dairy helps you trim calories. Sure, we all know that fat-free milk is a healthier choice than, say, gobs of whipped cream. But I found that most of my clients who were trying to lose weight inevitably had some "dairy creep" in their diet. This isn't surprising, given the enormous amounts of it oozing from every corner of our culture—things like cheese, sour cream, ice cream, even coffee drinks. A little here, a little there . . . can add up to a *lot* of calories. So let's get specific. To get into the slim zone, choose reduced-fat and fat-free dairy products in your 1-cup-a-day choice; these versions help keep saturated fat and calorie levels in check while still letting you enjoy the health and taste benefits of dairy products.

A lean and green diet does not include fatty dairy products like cream, cream cheese, butter, sour cream, and ice cream on a regular basis; at most, they should be considered splurges and eaten a few times a year. These foods are loaded with saturated fat and calories and are a fast track to the fat lane, the chronically ill lane, and statin land. They are high-carbon choices with high costs to your health and your waistline.

Reason #2: There are leaner and greener ways to bone up on calcium. It may surprise you to learn that you can meet your entire calcium needs without any dairy products whatsoever. In fact, more than 75 percent of the world's population is lactose intolerant, so they live quite well with little or no dairy products in their diets. It may also surprise you to learn that populations with the lowest intakes of calcium in the world (citizens of India and Japan have a daily intake of about 300 milligrams) have some of the lowest rates of hip fracture and osteoporosis, while people with some of the highest intakes (citizens of the United States and Finland have average intakes of at least 1,000 milligrams a day) also have some of the highest rates of osteoporosis.[1] We will get a bit more into the politics shortly, but one thing we do know is that three-quarters of the world's population have found ways to get adequate calcium in their diets without dairy, and you can, too.

CHEESE: A SPLURGE IN EVERY SENSE

You'll notice in your Lean and Green Prescription that you can have up to 5 ounces of cheese a month. If you're like most Americans, that's a big reduction, as well it should be. At roughly 100 calories an ounce, cheese is a splurge in every sense of the word.

It's time to start thinking of cheese as you would a rich dessert: a high-calorie, high-fat, but incredibly satisfying treat that you should eat only in small amounts a couple of times a month. Something to be savored and enjoyed, but less frequently and in smaller portions. (I know, trust me, cheese was one of my best pals; it is still around but has now become a more occasional friend.) It's amazing, but after a short adjustment, limiting your cheese consumption works and becomes super easy. You'll feel lighter and look better. Take those thoughtless cheese occasions out of your diet (on your sandwich, as an afternoon snack, left over from the snack put out at your child's playdate, at your book club when you've already eaten but it's just sitting there in front of you). Remember, *you can still have cheese*. Only now you are going to enjoy it in a more sustainable way.

If you're a die-hard cheese fan, you may be wondering how low-fat cheese shakes out. Personally and professionally, I am not a fan. Here is why: First, low-fat cheeses are still carbon intensive to produce because they are processed foods. Second, I find that for many people, they often don't seem to provide the same satiety that smaller portions of "the real thing" do. And third, they still contain calories, so unless you're still watching *portions* (which was difficult for many of my clients, who were tempted to eat more because it was low-fat), there's not necessarily a weight loss benefit.

If you prefer to use low-fat or fat-free cheese in your 5-ounce allotment, feel free to do so. But still keep it to 5 ounces if you want to get lean. Fat-free cheese may or may not be lower in calories, and weight is related to total calorie intake, not fat intake.

Now that you're a flexitarian, remember that you're *already* getting significantly more calcium by eating more tofu and beans. In addition to these, the nuts, seeds, and vegetables you'll be eating on the lean and green diet are going to go a long way toward meeting your calcium needs; add a glass of fortified rice milk or soymilk, plus a cup of dairy product, and you'll easily cruise to the finish line. Check out "Need Calcium? No Problem" on page 113 to see how easy it is to reach your daily calcium requirement (1,000 milligrams per day if you're age 19 to 50; 1,200 milligrams per day if you're over 50) without even touching a glass of milk, if you really want to be green. If you think that your diet may not be up to snuff when it comes to calcium, then you may want to consider taking a supplement that meets the guidelines suggested in Chapter 2.

Reason #3: Cutting back on dairy is critical to lightening your carbon load. As we've already discussed, beef and dairy products are the two highest-carbon ingredients in your diet. But if you want to harness the health benefits of live dairy foods, or if you are not feeling like you are able or willing to move to a completely vegan diet (which I personally am not, and many of my clients are not as well), the Lean and Green Prescription above brings you to a better balance. Following the prescription will make you a more conscious consumer of a high-carbon product. By targeting the *right* kinds of dairy products, in the right amounts, you can reap their health benefits and taste, and keep this additional delicious variety in your life but in a more sustainable way. It simplifies your life by giving you clear, limited choices. A win-win.

Dairy

At this point, you may be asking, "Well, why are you including dairy products at all if they're so bad for the planet?" It's a good question, and the answer takes us one step deeper into the powerful compounds that the right kinds of dairy can deliver for health. Aside from taste and enjoyment, and aside from a healthy dose of protein, calcium, and vitamins A and D (all of which you probably already know about), there are certain benefits that a daily serving of dairy is beautifully designed to provide. Here are some of the highlights.

LEAN BENEFITS

Conjugated linoleic acid (CLA) is a naturally occurring type of fat found primarily in products from grass-fed animals. Once far more

DOES MILK HELP YOU LOSE WEIGHT?

Those full-page ads sure make it sound easy and straightforward, don't they? "Drink Milk. Lose Weight." These headlines go on to claim that drinking 24 ounces in 24 hours on a low-calorie diet helps you lose weight faster than if you skip the milk.

But is it whitewashing? Probably. The dairy industry is quick to suggest that this finding is due to some special benefit that milk confers (such as speeding up metabolism or preventing fat storage). But whether or not three servings of dairy provides some advantage, or whether the dairy industry is milking the data, is still open to much debate. In fact, a lengthy 2008 review of 49 randomized clinical trials found that consuming calcium or dairy products doesn't help people lose weight or even maintain their current weight.[2] Dairy products compose a wide category that varies tremendously in nutrition profile (i.e., how can you give sweeping guidelines when cottage cheese, low-fat yogurt, and whole milk all have different nutrition profiles?). And within the nutrition community there is still much debate as to how much dairy you need.

As a dietitian, I can't help but notice that these studies have been funded by the dairy industry and that the lead researcher in many of these studies also happens to hold a patent on the calcium-and-weight-loss claim. What's more, if you actually read the nitty-gritty (which they know most people won't), the results don't sound nearly as revolutionary as the splashy ads would have you believe. The studies found that people who lost weight were following a reduced-calorie diet that included milk.[3] Big whoop. Anyone following a reduced-calorie diet is more likely to lose weight. Right now, there's not enough convincing evidence that milk is a silver (or white) bullet to weight loss. In my opinion, the only evidence that really seems worth extracting from these studies is the same old advice—reduce calories, lose weight. Period.

present in our hunter-gatherer diets, it's almost nonexistent in our processed-food, feedlot-fed culture, and there is a growing call from some physicians and naturopaths that this lack of CLA is part of the problem with our current industrial diet. Milk from grass-fed cows has been found to be up to four times higher in CLA than conventional milk and cheese.[4]

Let me stress here that I am a proponent of naturally occurring

NEED CALCIUM? NO PROBLEM[5]

FOOD	CALCIUM (MG)	FOOD	CALCIUM (MG)
1 cup nonfat organic yogurt	467	1 cup Swiss chard, boiled	102
½ cup tofu with calcium sulfate	434	2 Tbsp almond butter	86
3 oz sardines, canned with bones	325	1 cup butternut squash, cooked	84
1 cup organic fat-free milk	301	1 cup chickpeas	80
1 cup enriched soymilk	299	1 oz almonds	75
1 cup collard greens, boiled	266	1 cup broccoli, boiled	62
1 cup turnip greens, boiled	197		

CLA through foods rather than supplements. Often, what works in nature, through the vehicle of whole foods, doesn't translate (and may even have negative effects) when isolated, condensed into a pill, and put into someone's diet. All over the Internet and in supplement aisles, CLA supplements are widely touted as a weight loss wonder pill, or a tool to help maintain healthy glucose metabolism. And while there is some evidence that CLA helps fight fat and regulate glucose, there are also some inconsistent studies, so my suggestion is to seek to include natural CLA-rich foods in your diet instead of taking pills.[6] At the very least, you're relying on thousands of years of gastronomic tradition (which science often seems to find is the best way to eat—big surprise) to bring this nutrient back into your diet. Naturally occurring CLA may likely have health benefits without potential drawbacks; researchers in both France and Finland, for example, have found significantly lower rates of breast cancer in women with the highest intakes of naturally occurring CLA.[7]

A European team found that mothers consuming mostly organic milk and meat products have about 50 percent higher levels of CLA in their breast milk.[8] And those amazing French traditional cheeses have been found to have more than twice the levels of CLA (because the animals are raised on pastures) than conventional American cheese.[9] While CLA is certainly not a cure-all, the evidence suggests that naturally occurring CLA (as opposed to supplements) may offer real health benefits.

Want more good news about sustainable dairy choices? Research has found organic milk to contain up to 70 to 240 percent more omega-3s (and a much better ratio of omega-3 to omega-6) than conventional milk.[10] In fact, at the risk of sounding like I've just exited the *Sound of Music* tour, grass-fed milk offers a slew of benefits: up to 50 percent higher levels of vitamin E, 75 percent higher levels of beta-carotene, two to three times more antioxidants, and up to 200 percent more omega-3s (in the form of linolenic acid).[11] It would seem these nutrients swiftly vanish in the feedlot.

Another reason I recommend including some dairy products in your diet? Real, all-natural yogurt contains probiotics, which render it a health wonderfood. You see, in this era of "Hand-Sanitizer-Everywhere-You-Go" obsession with cleanliness (which is especially popular for the "moms toting tots" set, of which I've been a part the past 3 years), people seem to have forgotten that many bacteria are actually good for us, and a healthy part of our bodies and our lives.

The average healthy person has about 100 trillion bugs living in his or her gut. *Whoa. Bugs?* Yup, you read that right. Bugs. Probiotics literally means "for life," and it refers to the good, healthy, friendly bacteria that thrive in your gut and help keep "bad" bugs in check. If you think of the worst case of traveler's diarrhea you've ever had, you can pretty quickly imagine what happens when "bad"

LOOK FOR THE SEAL

Look for yogurt with the National Yogurt Association's "Live and Active Cultures" (LAC) seal to be sure you're getting the right amount of live cultures. Labels these days can be misleading; all yogurt begins with cultures, but you want to be sure you're getting a brand that reintroduces probiotics after pasteurization. The LAC seal signals that the product contains at least 100 million live cultures for each gram of yogurt, which is a good benchmark to aim for. The two most common probiotics added to dairy are *lactobacillus acidophilus* and *B. bifidum*, but there are others as well.

GREEN YOUR PANTRY: PROJECT PANTRY PURGE

■ Purge your fridge of the following high-calorie, high-carbon "creams": heavy cream and half-and-half, ice cream, sour cream, and cream cheese. They can have about 100 calories a tablespoon, consisting mostly of artery-clogging saturated fat. Yikes!

■ Stash your butter in the freezer so you'll have it handy for occasional baking but won't be tempted on a daily basis.

■ For a cooler indulgence, choose a 100 percent fruit sorbet or one of the amazing soy-based frozen desserts available instead of ice cream.

■ Pick a smarter spread: Use all-natural almond or peanut butter instead of cream cheese or butter.

■ Use a few slices of avocado in place of sour cream.

■ Start your day with freshly brewed green tea instead of a high-calorie coffee confection.

■ Include organic, all-natural, low-fat or nonfat yogurt that's packed with good-for-you probiotics to help you get on the fast track to healthy and lean. To control calories and carbon, buy plain and then mix in your own fruit, honey, or sugar; you will likely add a lot less than many of the flavored commercial brands.

■ Stock your fridge or pantry with soymilk or rice milk. Soymilk is available nearly everywhere regular milk is sold these days. Refrigerated soymilk, which comes in lots of flavors, is found right next to the regular milk in the dairy section (and has the same packaging, so recycling's a cinch). There's also boxed soy- and rice milk that's shelf stable (which you pop in the fridge after opening), usually located in the cereal aisle or the natural foods section.

■ Log on to www.realmilk.com to locate the best sources of organic, grass-fed milk in your area. Move to these products as you continue your shift to lighter living.

bugs get the upper hand. But there may be more subtle ways that our bodies are out of whack because we no longer get enough of the "good" bacteria in our diet; things like allergies, eczema, fatigue, yeast infections, and general intestinal "distress" all may be connected in some ways to a lack of a healthy gut balance.

While probiotics are sometimes overhyped these days (they are being added to all sorts of food products, which are then being hocked as "health food"), here are some facts. "Good bugs" (or healthy bacteria) help fight inflammation, aid with nutrient absorption and the production of certain vitamins (such as vitamin K), help maintain a favorable pH balance in your gut, reduce the risk of vaginal yeast infections and urinary tract infections, and keep the lining of your gut working effectively. And a healthy, functioning gut is one of the most important aspects of a strong, powerful, well-working immune system. Antibiotics, diet, stress, a bout of traveler's diarrhea, even aging can all interfere with this balance, so it's a good idea to replenish your body from the inside out with healthy bugs.

While the idea that tossing back a few billion bacteria a day can do wonders for your health may seem hard to swallow, traditional folklore in many parts of the world venerated these fermented foods as vital to good health and longevity. Yogurt in Eastern Europe, for example, and miso in Japan have long been touted for their healing properties. And when I worked as a caterer in Boston during graduate school, many of the newly arrived young Irish women I worked with told me stories of how at their homes in Ireland, their parents would set aside some of the fresh milk each morning, put it in a bowl, and leave it out on the counter all day long; it was then used as buttermilk the following day. While this last one is probably enough to give food sanitation experts heart palpitations, these are all traditional examples of good bugs at work.

While the rest of our sterilized food supply has lost many of the naturally occurring "bugs," there's a growing body of science to suggest that there may just be some truth to the folklore. Probiotics have been shown to shorten the course of diarrhea in infants and children, and to help minimize and neutralize the symptoms of irritable bowel syndrome (IBS).[12] And a dose of probiotics may also help "reboot" your gut after a bout of traveler's diarrhea or a dose of antibiotics (which, of course, wipes out the healthy bugs along with the ones that are making you sick). Probiotics can also inhibit the growth of *Candida albicans,* which may be helpful in preventing yeast infections in women.[13] And the great news is, unlike most supplements or drugs, probiotics can safely be included as a healthy addition to nearly everyone's diet (one possible exception is if you are immunocompromised, such as if you have cancer or are HIV positive, so be sure to check with your doctor first).

GREEN BENEFITS

There's no getting around it: Skipping dairy altogether is greener for the planet. Moving to a diet with fewer animal products is one of the most powerful things you can do for your health and your contribution to global warming. It would be irresponsible for me to suggest anything else.

There's a lot more left behind than just that milk mustache. Cows create some of the most powerful greenhouse gases and are still a "middleman" (or middle cow) in the energy cycle. Cheese, milk, and yogurt of course *come* from animals, so they're heavy carbon hitters, linked with agriculture and all of those issues we covered in Part II when you began your flexitarian lifestyle. Because of this, moving from a typical American diet to a vegan one will do more to cut your carbon footprint than switching from an SUV to a hybrid, cutting about *half a ton* per year more carbon from your footprint than would just swapping rides.[14]

Even if ol' Daisy lives right next door to you, even if you *own* Daisy yourself, while you've gone local (good for you), you still have a few issues you can't skirt around. No matter where they live, the US Department of Energy estimates that dairy cows are responsible for about 30 percent of the total cow burps and farts that are adding powerful global warming gases to the planet (methane is 20 times more powerful at trapping heat than carbon, and nitrous oxide is a whopping 300 times more powerful).[15] An average cow can add about

HOW TINY TASTES CAN ADD UP . . . TO BIG CALORIES

"Why can't I lose weight?" "I never snack between meals. . . . I know I'm not perfect, but I really don't eat that much junk."

	CALORIES	TOTAL FAT (W/SAT FAT)
Monday: Oops! Forgot to ask them to hold the cheese on your sandwich.	114	9 grams (6 g saturated)
Tuesday: Helped yourself to a bit of cheese at book club, after all, it's just a small nibble—not like you ate the whole thing: 2 ounces brie cheese.	190	16 grams (10 g saturated)
Wednesday: Gobbled the last couple bites of your child's lunch as you left the restaurant— 2 tablespoons of sour cream on that quesadilla.	51	5 grams (3 g saturated)
Thursday: At that morning meeting, tore off a small piece of bagel because the boss was doing it, too—2 tablespoons of cream cheese on that morning bagel.	101	10 grams (6 g saturated)
Friday: At the mall and feeling parched; decide to split a 16-ounce vanilla frappuccino with your teenage daughter. Hey, isn't splitting a great strategy? Your share:	215	7 gram (4.5 g saturated)
Sunday: At the market, help yourself to a free "teensie" sample of ice cream: 1/4 cup Häagen-Dazs vanilla ice cream	135	9 grams (5.5 g saturated)

Weekly Total: 806 calories. Monthly Total: just under about 1 pound. Yearly total: 11 pounds.
References:
USDA CALCULATOR: http://www.nal.usda.gov/fnic/foodcomp/search/index.html
Häagen-Dazs website: http://www.haagendazs.com/products/product.aspx?id=104
http://www.haagendazs.com/products/product.aspx?id=314 (Accessed June 5, 2008)
http://www.starbucks.com/retail/nutrition_beverage_detail.asp

500 liters each day of methane to your local air. Nice. A local cow still eats. A local cow still poops. A local cow still requires water. All of this means lots of fossil fuel to manage.

So that's why it's really important to take a bit less, to be sure you buy from farmers committed to sustainable practices, and swap some of your dairy for soy, which is easier than ever to do these days. Today, even your barista and local ice cream joint are likely to offer soymilk or soy ice cream, which packs the fun and flavor of dairy but without the global warming underbelly of dairy. In the next chapter, we'll fully address the "Is localism better?" question, but if you really can't stand the idea of going a day without dairy, let me just continue by pointing out a few reasons why local is worth it if you can find it, even if "local" is a bit relative.

First, local dairy is fresher dairy. It will log fewer miles and is much more likely to get to you sooner, which means better taste and a greater preservation of the more volatile nutrients (such as riboflavin). It also means less time idling in a chilly, greenhouse-gas-pumping refrigerator. So going local will likely help trim some of this additional carbon load.

Second, local dairy may also be less expensive. My in-laws, who live in rural Connecticut on teacher salaries, have an amazing network of local dairy, pork, beef, and chicken all through farmer friends of theirs. Some of these are even organic (although not officially certified). My other in-laws, in upstate New York and living on fixed teacher pensions, amazingly have the same type of network. Most of their friends eat this way because it's *cheaper,* not because it's organic or better for the planet. With the rising cost of basic food staples a real concern for people all across the country, there can be a powerful overlap between eating and sourcing locally and saving some money.

I point this out to emphasize that organic and local are not the exclusive domain of the wealthy with unlimited means. Often those in more rural settings can actually find access to high-quality farm products more easily and at a reasonable price, so be a sleuth in your area and see what's happening locally. This is one of the pluses of our strong dairy heritage in America, so leverage it and cut the food miles and likely the cost. And if you buy from local dairies, you help keep these farmers in business.

So my recommendation is this: If you can only afford limited organics, make sure milk is on that list, especially if you have children. Conventional milk often contains recombinant bovine growth hormone, or rBGH (also called recombinant bovine somatotropin, or rBST). This is a synthetic hormone that, when injected into cows, can increase milk production by 10 to 20 percent. Because of the spiderweb of health and politics, milk that contains this hormone is not required to be labeled, so unless your milk is organic, assume that it does. You may be able to find dairies that, due to FDA regulations (again, protecting business first), indicate that they do not use rBGH, and their products will bear a statement that begins with "The FDA has found no significant difference between milk . . . ," so at the very least, look for milk that touts this sort of label. But rBGH is banned in Australia, Canada, New Zealand, Japan, and the European Union. And the UN Food Standards Body and the World Trade Organization (WTO) both refused to endorse it.

As a nutritionist, the concern I have with rBGH is that milk from cows injected with it has higher levels of insulin-like growth factor 1 (IGF-1). IGF-1 is a powerful steroidlike hormone that is identical in both cows and humans; it is important in childhood growth and may also speed the aging process. While the FDA and Monsanto (the company that makes rBGH) contend that because the natural IGF-1 present in milk is virtually identical to the IGF-1 that shows up in milk of cows treated with rBGH, there's no health risk. I am not convinced. Several studies have found that higher IGF-1 levels might be linked to prostate and breast cancer.[17] While IGF-1 levels are impacted by several factors, including weight, physical fitness, and heredity, the truth is there is still no definitive data to prove whether getting more IGF-1 in your milk is harmful or not. So why risk it? There are so many green advantages to organic that it is a no-brainer as far as I'm concerned, and critical if you are giving milk to your children.

Is organic greener? Up to the farm gate, yes. Organic dairy cuts out a major piece of the greenhouse gas puzzle—the pesticides and fertilizers. According to a UK report, it takes about three times as much energy to produce a liter of conventional milk as it does to produce a liter of organic.[18] However, if that organic butter is flown to you from Europe, or that organic milk is shipped, chilled, across the country to you, those carbon advantages can disappear in a haze of fumes. So drink like a local.

Okay, now that I've beaten that cow to death, let me briefly tell you why I think eggs are so great.

Eggs: All They're Cracked Up to Be

As I just said, eggs are pretty darn great. And unless you have food allergies to eggs, you can be eating about five or six local

WHAT ABOUT CHOLESTEROL?

Concerned about cholesterol? Then check with your MD first. But make sure your doctor is up to snuff on the latest. Old school: Eggs are bad. New school? Eggs are fine in moderation and aren't responsible for raising triglycerides and cholesterol, so you don't need to take eggs off of your plate.[19] (I've found that some of my clients seem to be working with cardiologists who for whatever reason haven't really heard the latest.) A Harvard study published in 1999 that looked at 120,000 men and women found that an egg a day over the long term isn't likely to raise blood cholesterol. *The Harvard Medical School Guide to Healthy Eating* concluded, "No research has ever shown that people who eat more eggs have more heart attacks than people who eat few eggs."[20] Rather, the real villain in heart disease is saturated fat, which is found in foods such as whole milk, meat, cheese, ice cream, and butter. So go on, there's no need to order up your eggs with a side of guilt anymore.

eggs per week (or ideally, organic and omega-3 fortified eggs if you can find them). By now, I know you're an expert on why organic and local matter, to both your health and the planet. The good news is that chickens are pretty green; in fact, they're one of the greenest animals in terms of manure waste and inputs.

At the risk of sounding like I've been hit over the head with my frying pan, let me assure you this is the nutritionist in me talking: Eggs are cheap and abundant, can be served up a million different ways with minimal cooking skills, contain all nine essential amino acids, and receive top ratings for protein quality. Loaded with B vitamins and folate, eggs are also rich in choline (great for brain functioning and for healthy cell membranes) and the antioxidants lutein and zeaxanthin, which help protect eyes from macular degeneration by filtering out harmful UV wavelengths. And naturopaths and holistic nutritionists say that the sulfur in eggs helps you radiate beauty because it promotes healthy hair and nails. Beautiful.

If you happen to have a very local egg source (a neighbor's coop or a nearby farm), it could be a great way to get amazingly fresh eggs for a steal. Even if you live in a city, you may be surprised at what you can find.

I continue to hear stories from people, whether in cities or rural areas, who have stumbled across a great "find" of one sort of food or another, near them, in an unexpected way. So start looking, and you may be amazed at what you discover.

Not only do super-fresh eggs have a wonderful taste, but they remove a significant part of the fossil fuel chain as well. In addition, if you can afford them, omega-3 fortified eggs will get you even more of the heart-healthy fats. Truly free-range chickens are also apt to have higher levels of omega-3 in their egg yolks. Otherwise, chickens are the greenest animal to be using in the food chain—and a healthy, happy chicken can go on to lay eggs for a long time.

TAKE ACTION NOW

SWAP OUT HIGH-FAT DAIRY FROM YOUR DAILY FARE.

- Switch from 1 cup of whole milk to 1 cup of fat-free a day and lose 70 calories in 1 day, an amount that can help you shed 7 pounds in a year.

- Skip that slice of cheese (140 calories) on your daily sandwich and lose 14 pounds in a year.

- Wake up with freshly brewed green tea instead of a 12-ounce latte (made with 2 percent milk, 150 calories) and lose 15.6 pounds in a year.

- Got a sustainable snack? Slather roasted red pepper or white bean dip on whole grain crackers for a satisfying snack that's leaner and greener than cheese slices.

- Spread mashed avocado or hummus on sandwiches instead of cheese for a tasty, nutritious spread.

- Show-stopping salads: Shower almonds, pistachios, sunflower or pumpkin seeds, or dried cranberries on your salad instead of cheese for a greener bite.

- Substitute fat-free refried beans or mashed, soft tofu instead of cheese in enchiladas and tacos.

GET THE BIGGEST BANG FOR YOUR BUCK.

- Select cheese with powerful flavor, such as authentic Parmigiano-Reggiano or extra-sharp Cheddar. Smaller amounts still pack powerful flavor.

EAT LIKE A EUROPEAN.

- Instead of serving cheese as an appetizer when everyone's starving and likely to shovel in way too much way too fast, serve it after the meal for dessert. Pair it with seasonal fruits like berries in summer, or dried fruit and nuts in winter.

- Insist on quality. Cheese sauces, "zappable cheese products" meant for the microwave, are apt to pack on calories and carbon with little nutrition. Choose the high-quality stuff, and savor it.

CHAPTER 9

PRODUCE

❝Imagine for a moment if we once again knew, strictly as a matter of course, these few unremarkable things: What it is we're eating. Where it comes from. How it found its way to our table. And what, in a true accounting, it really cost.❞

—Michael Pollan, *The Omnivore's Dilemma*

YOUR LEAN AND GREEN PRESCRIPTION
1½ cups fruit and 3–4 cups vegetables every day

(Power fruits and veggies pack lots of color: reds, orange, dark greens, blue/purple)

INCLUDE
All fresh fruits and vegetables (especially those that are in season and deeply colored)

Fresh leafy greens and salad greens (especially darker colors) and fresh and dried mushrooms

Frozen "naked" fruits and vegetables (no sauces or syrups)

GREENER
Something grown in season locally, or that you grow yourself

Up to the farm gate, organic is greener. Go organic to the extent possible, but balanced with prudent transportation.

Try to minimize overpackaged products to the extent that you can while still sticking with your Prescription.

LIMIT (STILL SUPER HEALTHY BUT MAY COME IN A HIGHER CALORIE/CARBON PACKAGE)
Up to 6 ounces 100 percent fruit or vegetable juice

¼ cup dried fruit

Canned tomatoes, artichokes, olives, roasted peppers, and pumpkin

AVOID
Any juice or juice blend that isn't 100 percent fruit or vegetable

Dried fruit with added oils or sweeteners

All other canned produce, especially those with added salt or in syrups/sauces

Fruit that has been flown on an airplane. (Typically that can include pineapples and other tropical fruits, as well as berries in wintertime. Ask your produce manager.)

If your diet consists mostly of lifeless, heavily processed and refined foods, odds are you, too, will feel lifeless. On the other hand, if your diet includes lots of vibrant foods teeming with nutrition and powerful enzymes, you too will feel more vibrant and alive. It's that simple.

Many of my clients share the same problem: They simply don't eat enough of these foods that can make them feel good, relying instead on "convenience," ready-to-eat, overly processed junk. They don't make the connection between what they're putting into their bodies and what they're getting in return.

Why am I telling you all of this now? Because this is the chapter where you truly make it happen. Here is where you begin shifting your plate to start experiencing health at the highest level. Here is where you discover the abundance of food that you can eat, that you *should* eat, while slimming down. Here is where you see firsthand how the right food choices can dramatically help the body heal from years (possibly decades) of bad food choices.

While all of my clients have different goals (an athlete seeks performance, a baby boomer wants to shed her "menopot" belly, a new mom wants to lose the baby weight), at the end of the day most of us are looking for the same thing—to feel and look our best. And the amount of produce you choose to include in your diet is the single biggest step you will take toward the body that you want.

In this era of quick fixes, pills and potions, of wanting to lose 10 pounds by last Tuesday, the immense power of plant foods is overlooked by most of us. But make no mistake. The produce aisle is where the power foods sit in the supermarket. If they represent an easy, low-tech, immediate way to begin creating better health and weight for yourself, they also offer an immediate, low-tech way to curb America's massive global emissions coming from our food supply. Healing in every sense.

So eat more. A lot more. Starting now.

LEAN BENEFITS

I get it all the time. When I am asked by clients or the media about which nutrients they should be pursuing, they look expectantly at me, imagining I am going to send them to the supplement aisle for some new exotic herb or undiscovered wonder pill, or to perhaps suggest that they subsist exclusively on cabbage soup and cayenne pepper. When I tell them to hit the produce aisle and load up on a variety of colors, they seem bored and deflated. They know *that,* but surely isn't there something else? Something faster, easier, and, well, *sexier* than that?

In a nutshell, nope. And deep down, if you're like most of my clients, you already know that. But you can hope, can't you? Sure, but remember that hope is not a strategy. Not for changing our health, and certainly not for fixing our climate crisis. Eating lots of wonderful produce, on the other hand, is.

Because you already know that fruits and veggies help you slim down due to their high-fiber/low-calorie combination (and who doesn't want to be able to eat more and still weigh less?), let's focus on a few other ways that produce creates a beautiful life, starting today.

When you pack your plate with a variety of colors, it's like hitting Mother Nature's pharmacy. And I'm talking about protection that goes way beyond things such as vitamin C for enhanced immunity.

I'll admit that a lot of the rhetoric around fruits and veggies is focused on things like reducing risk of heart attack and stroke, which to many people may seem far off and vaguely boring at this point in their lives. So let's talk about some of the short-term, more immediate pressing concerns, such as wrinkles. An international team of researchers who studied people from several countries (which means several different eating patterns) found that in each population, foods such as red meat, whole milk, sodas, and pastries were associated with significantly more skin damage, while people with the most wrinkle-free skin regularly ate more produce, especially richly colored produce.[1] Their results weren't altogether surprising. Fruits and veggies are loaded with antioxidants, and most skin damage is caused by oxidative stress that occurs when sunlight hits the skin. A lean and green diet that fights wrinkles, too? Sign me up.

Another surprising effect of a produce-rich diet? Keeping your lean muscle mass intact, which helps keep your metabolism burning

10 WAYS TO PACK IN THE PRODUCE

■ Consider produce a nonnegotiable starting point for every meal and snack. Pack fruit into smoothies, tuck veggies onto sandwiches, serve last night's extra roasted veggies alongside a scrambled egg or in a frittata, nosh on fruit for a midmorning snack.

■ Follow the color rule: three colors on your plate at meals, two colors for snacks.

■ Catch up at dinner. Heap at least two vegetables onto your plate. Learn an easy surefire prep method, like roasting in the oven with olive oil (or tossing on the grill in summer), so you can't make excuses such as, "I don't know how to prepare them."

■ If you see it, you'll eat it: Spend 2 minutes getting healthy picks at the ready and in plain sight when you open the fridge. Sliced bell peppers and cucumber with hummus, for example, are much easier to grab when they're all set. Marinate some meaty mushrooms in your favorite dressings and toss on the grill as a super-healthy addition to your lean and green cuisine.

■ Eat with the seasons. In winter, have pureed butternut squash soup with half a sandwich for lunch; in summer, feast on fresh local berries after supper, or pop local cherry tomatoes as a snack. The food will taste better and appeal to your natural cravings.

■ Be picky at the supermarket. Use some of your newfound food dollars to buy the best quality you can afford—your reward will be better taste.

■ Stock your freezer with your favorite naked frozen fruits and veggies to help you in a pinch.

■ Use local dried fruit or small amounts of 100 percent fruit or vegetable juice to sneak in a serving when fresh isn't an option.

■ If you're in the winter doldrums and local is scarce, loosen your notion of local a bit and keep eating those fruits and veggies. Find some produce with longer growing seasons—like mushrooms—to help you in the colder months.

■ For a super-easy, no-brainer way to start, find the current season in the back of this book and follow the week of meals starting on page 228. I've done the thinking and planning for you.

at a higher rate. Fruits and vegetables are chock-full of potassium, which experts have long known helps cut your risk of stroke, bone loss, and kidney stones and *also* stems the muscle loss that typically occurs every year with age.

A 2008 study in the *American Journal of Clinical Nutrition* measured urinary potassium levels and found that subjects with the highest potassium intakes had a higher percentage of lean muscle tissue, while those with lower potassium levels had significantly less lean muscle mass.[2]

Why is potassium protective against losing muscle? The typical American diet is rich in acid-producing foods such as meat and cereals. Over time, these foods can gradually disrupt the body's natural acid-base balance, which triggers a muscle-wasting response as the body attempts to buffer the excess acid. Fruits and vegetables are high in potassium, which is a wonderful neutralizer because it produces alkaline in the body, which in turn helps keep your lean muscle tissue intact.

Lean muscle tissue is like a furnace that is cooking away at a higher temperature than body fat ever does, so it requires significantly more calories just to maintain. That's why keeping your lean muscle tissue intact is a key strategy in being able to eat more food and still lose weight.

Unfortunately, when you look at the statistics, what passes as "vegetables" for most of us in America is, let's be honest, comical even to a non-nutritionist: One-third of all vegetables consumed in the United States are in the form of french fries, potato chips, and iceberg lettuce, hardly nutritional powerhouses. The food industry would like you to believe that that thin purplish line squeaking out from a breakfast cereal bar qualifies as "fruit." And remember when the Reagan administration tried to convince us that ketchup was a vegetable?

So remember this easy rule: *Color is key*. Pack color into your diet, starting today. Make sure you don't have a "white diet" that's loaded with white bread and rice, sugary breakfast cereals, mashed potatoes and french fries, and iceberg lettuce. Not only will you have awful constipation (there's little fiber in those foods), but you're also missing out on the power of color to keep you healthy.

THE POWER OF COLOR[3]

COLOR	FOUND IN	BENEFITS
RED	Strawberries, cherries, watermelons, tomatoes, pink grapefruit	**LYCOPENE:** A member of the carotenoid family, it acts as a powerful free-radical scavenger and may greatly cut your risk of developing prostate and lung cancer.
	Pomegranates, cranberries	**ELLAGIC ACID:** Shown to reduce esophageal and colon tumors; appears to slow down the growth rate of and even trigger *apoptosis* ("cell death") in cancer cells.
GREEN	Broccoli, Brussels sprouts, Swiss chard, kale, turnip greens	**LUTEIN AND ZEAXANTHIN:** Helps protect the eyes from age-related macular degeneration, the leading cause of vision loss in Americans 60 years and older.
ORANGE	Carrots, pumpkins, sweet potatoes, mangoes, apricots	**BETA-CAROTENE:** This antioxidant has been shown to cut cancer and stroke risk, as well as help raise immunity ability.
BLUE/PURPLE	Berries, grapes	**RESVERATROL:** Helps keep artery walls healthy and reduces the risk of stroke and heart attack.
WHITE	Garlic, onions, apples	**QUERCETIN:** One of the flavonoids, it mops up free radicals, has been shown to kill the herpes virus, cuts the incidence of heart attack, and is a strong antiviral and anti-inflammatory.

Now let's get specific. While *all* produce, pale and vibrant alike, has something to offer, I tell my clients to aim for around three or more colors at each meal, and two or more at each snack. That way you are sure to get a healthy cocktail of nature's protection every time you eat. Of course, we're talking about naturally occurring pigments (i.e., blueberries versus blue-colored ketchup, dark leafy greens as opposed to a green-chocolate-covered candy). You can even count the darker hues in whole grains, beans, mushrooms, legumes—even that daily glass of red wine—in this "color count."

In addition to staying leaner and developing fewer wrinkles, take a look at the table on page 129 to see a few of the other ways eating more fruits and vegetables can help you experience health at the highest level.

Before we get to the green benefits, I'd like to make two quick comments about your Prescription. First, I'm sure you noticed that I included all fresh fruits and vegetables in the leanest category. I'm not going to quibble over a few calories between produce types, especially given the power of the whole package, so keep it simple for yourself. Trust me, Americans are not the fattest people on the planet because we're overdoing it on fruits and veggies.

Second, you'll recall that I mentioned minimizing packaging to the extent that you can while still keeping your Prescription. Here's why: The produce aisle has exploded with different packages of precut fruits and vegetables, which ultimately has made it easier for many busy Americans to eat them. In my opinion, this trend is ultimately a good thing for the planet because it's good for human health, even if it does come with the burden of higher packaging in the short term. However, the added convenience does come with a higher grocery bill (sometimes much higher), so if you have the time to prepare them, buy whole fruits and vegetables whenever possible.

So now that you know your basic Prescription from a lean standpoint, let's take a closer look at some of the issues that go into how "green" your pack of pickled peppers may or may not be.

GREEN BENEFITS

In the spring of 2005, I was in the Loire Valley in France, planning a conference on childhood obesity and school lunches that I hosted with Field to Plate in 2006. We had stopped at this charming little café, and our host Phillipe insisted that we order the local *spécialité*, fresh cream of mushroom soup with thyme.

It is not an exaggeration to say that each spoonful was pure heaven. One taste and I sank into idiocy as the intense, meaty mushroom flavor floating in a sea of cream washed over each ecstatic tastebud. It was nothing like the quivering tower of gray stuff I'd seen plopped in a pan and heated for lunch when I was younger. Never, I realized, had I actually tasted cream of mushroom soup until that very moment.

"Phillipe," I cooed, "this is incredible! Are these mushrooms local?"

"*Non,*" he said brusquely, with a wave of his hand. "They are from two villages away."

Two villages away. That pretty much sums up the difference in expectations of "local" between the French and the Americans when it comes to food.

Welcome to the next part of living a leaner and greener lifestyle—eating like a "locavore" for a couple of meals each week. As a locavore, you're going to start tapping into more foods that are being grown or produced near you. You will *make the season the foundation of your fresh food choices,* which is guaranteed to freshen up your cart with some new options, give you more variety throughout the year, and help shake you out of the shopping rut that we all get in from time to time. Most important, it means you are about to move to your healthiest, slimmest self while thinning that haze of carbon emissions wafting up from your global shopping cart. Because here is another key overlap in the new lean and green cuisine: One of the strongest calls coming from food energy experts is to diversify what we grow. And one of the best dietary strategies to maximize health is to eat a wide variety of foods. Diversification of the American diet away from a corn-centric ingredient list (and all its thousands of derivations) offers a healthy, fresh start on both fronts.

So, back to the produce. In order to help you see the many levels of leaner and greener choices, let me be clear: From a weight standpoint, an apple is (more or less) an apple no matter where it's from. And the *most* important thing for losing weight is that you actually eat your fruits and vegetables rather than become paralyzed by the ethical maze of which choice is the absolute best. I have seen many clients fall into that trap, and believe me, all this does is prevent you from moving toward your goals.

As I've said, the carbon savings are big when you move to plants; produce requires an average of 2 calories of energy to

FRESH, FROZEN, OR CANNED?

As I wrote this book, dozens of people offered up hundreds of questions to see where their favorite foods would land on the lean and green scale. Overall, their questions were extremely helpful in letting me see things through a client's perspective, but this particular question was perhaps the most vexing.

From a "lean" lens, the answer is easy. Truly fresh produce contains the vibrancy of nutrients and antioxidants and phytochemicals in a way that frozen and canned cannot wholly recapture. This is one of the pluses of rediscovering local foods when you can, so stick to fresh produce as much as possible. But "fresh" broccoli that has limped to your market from another country and is drooping on the shelf is apt to have lost some or most of its nutrients. In that case, hit the freezer aisle.

"Naked" frozen fruits and vegetables are a very good second choice, and if the "fresh" options look less than stellar, the frozen varieties will most likely offer even more nutrients. Technology today makes it easy to lock in much of the nutrition and powerful plant compounds, and frozen is a lifesaver when you're time strapped or can't hit the market. It's also a great way to eat on a budget, so if you can't afford to eat fresh, hit the freezer aisle to reap the benefits. Choose naked fruits and vegetables with no sauces or syrups, so you can control what goes on your plate.

For the most part, limit canned produce to the extent that your budget allows. (I made a few exceptions in your Prescription where the health benefits are worth it.) In general, seek canned produce that comes in water, versus syrups, oils, or sauces that can add calories and sodium.

---

produce 1 calorie of food, while animal proteins require 20 to 80 calories of energy for 1 calorie of food.[4]

So just what kinds of savings are we talking about? A 2008 study in the *Journal of Environmental Science and Technology* determined that simply switching from meat to vegetables for 1 day per week shaves off the equivalent of driving 1,160 miles per year.[5] If every American did that, 1.7 billion gallons of gasoline would be saved. If we all strived for local foods, the savings would be even more.

As you've probably noticed, supermarkets these days seem to

In terms of green, hands down, growing your own garden is the greenest of all. After that, local and seasonal is a very good bet. And after that, it gets fuzzy fast.

If you want to talk about the carbon merits of frozen versus canned, you can quickly get bogged down in a haze of mind-boggling "if, but" scenarios that would tax King Solomon. I'll show you how easy it can be to do that with this little ditty of consciousness (this is *you*, sitting in the store, agonizing over the "best" choice) . . .

"Well, canning is about 10 times as energy intensive as fresh, but then again a canned product has a long shelf life and can be kept at room temperature. And if I recycle the can, well, the carbon footprint will be lower as it offsets the energy involved in making the can. But if I don't recycle it, hmmm, it will be higher. The final carbon footprint of frozen produce (which is less energy intensive than canning at the onset but more energy intensive than fresh) depends on how long it sits in my freezer until it's used. But there's a lot less packaging per ounce of food, so that is greener . . . but, what's this, my organic frozen broccoli is from *China*?!? And oh no, this supermarket has its freezer aisles sitting open wafting greenhouse gases up into the air . . . "

See what I mean? It can start to make the tax code seem simple in comparison, and the last thing you need in your hectic life is paralysis by analysis. So here's my best advice: Don't worry about it. There are more important areas of your diet where you can have a much bigger impact on calories and carbon (e.g., meat, dairy). If you see a glaring carbon error, by all means avoid it. And stick with what's best from a nutrition standpoint: fresh and frozen.

offer virtually the same snapshot of produce options regardless of season or geography. Gone are the days of anticipating the first strawberries of the summer or fresh-picked local corn. Instead, our globalized supermarkets provide us with a truly movable feast of all produce, all the time. As a result, our produce has become more drenched in fossil fuel than it is in calories or nutrients. And here are a few of the reasons why.

- Consumers demand the same supply of food year-round independent of season and locale.

- Mega chain retailers and large supermarkets use centralized processing, packaging, and distribution centers. All of this adds carbon. Often, food that is grown locally isn't even sold locally.

- Labor in developing countries is much cheaper, which means lower-cost produce for you.

- Highly perishable foods grown in warmer climates are sometimes shipped in airplanes to minimize hold time.

- Our demand for precut, pre-done, ready-to-go everything has upped the packaging requirements.

All of this adds petroleum and food miles to our plates.

While rising fuel costs may change this (as it makes less and less economic sense to grow food in far-flung places and then ship it around the globe), as of now, most of our produce not only racks up frequent-flier miles but also fossil fuel. Consider that iceberg lettuce imported to the United Kingdom from the United States by plane requires 127 calories of energy to transport 1 calorie of lettuce across the Atlantic. For every mile traveled by an 18-wheeler to haul our food around the United States, 3.74 pounds of carbon dioxide are

GREEN CUISINE MADE EASY[6]

Stumped as to what grows when? Here's a quick primer appropriate to most regions of the country. Check with your local state extension agency to see exactly what's available to you.

SPRING	SUMMER	FALL	WINTER
Asparagus	Berries	Apples	Beets
Greens/lettuces	Cantaloupes and watermelons	Asian pears	Cabbage
Peas	Corn	Cranberries	Brussels sprouts
Peaches	Bell peppers	Potatoes and sweet potatoes	Parsnips
Morel mushrooms	Tomatoes	Onions	Citrus
Spinach	Plums	Turnips	Winter squashes

emitted. So driving one truck of strawberries from California to New York puts more than 11,000 pounds of carbon dioxide into the atmosphere—more than 4 ounces of carbon dioxide for each 12-ounce box of strawberries.[7]

CHECKING THE FOOD ODOMETER:
HOW FAR DOES YOUR PRODUCE TRAVEL?

The following table shows the average distance produce was found to travel by truck in a 2003 study by Iowa State University. The researchers found that by sourcing locally, they were able to shave the fuel bill down to *about ½₂₇ of the distance* from farm to plate, reducing the average food miles from 1,494 miles to just 56 miles. If just 10 percent of Iowans' food was actually grown within Iowa, researchers concluded, the annual fuel savings would be between 295,000 to 350,000 gallons of gas, and the greenhouse gas savings between 7 million and 7.9 million pounds.[8]

Definitely food for thought.

FOOD	DISTANCE	FOOD	DISTANCE
Grapes (table)	2,143 miles	Peas, green	2,102 miles
Broccoli	2,095 miles	Spinach	2,086 miles
Asparagus	1,671 miles	Strawberries	1,944 miles
Apples	1,555 miles		

By now, you may be scratching your head and wondering, So is local food more energy efficient? Here's the surprise answer: not necessarily. But you should still try to eat local anyway, as much as your local growing season allows, for a strong lean and green overlap. I'll tell you why shortly, but for now, let's look at some of the reasons localism isn't a silver bullet for a smaller carbon footprint.

While localism no doubt cuts food miles, the absolute carbon advantages of localism depend on where you live, on the time of year, and on the specific foods in question. Tomatoes grown in a greenhouse locally, for instance, may actually be more energy intensive to produce than tomatoes grown somewhere warmer and shipped to you.

While "food miles" is one marker of carbon footprint, there are others that may be bigger; how food is produced and packaged and stored, for instance, seem to matter as much, if not more. A 2008 study found that transportation created only about 11 percent of the total greenhouse gas emissions (about 8.1 metric tons) in an average US household's "food footprint," while agriculture and industry practices accounted for 83 percent.[9] They also found that switching to a totally local diet is the equivalent of saving about 1,000 miles from the distance you drive your car each year, and that much bigger, more significant carbon savings were to be had by cutting back on meat and dairy.[10] (As we already saw, simply moving 1 day a week from meat to plants yields bigger savings.)

"The argument that reducing food miles decreases fossil fuel consumption appears so obvious, so intuitively logical, that it would seem anyone who questions it must be insane, work for Exxon Mobil, or live in the food-exporting nation of New Zealand," noted one plucky journalist.[11]

Funny he should say that, because in fact it *was* New Zealand who fought back against this localized thing and produced some data about lamb production (which I shared with you in Chapter 5). Another hole in the theory came when a 2005 study found that the Kiwis' production of Braeburn apples outyielded German Braeburn orchards by a factor of two, for a net energy efficiency of 25 percent.[12] Clearly, there may be some cases where natural geography creates a smaller carbon footprint.

WHY DOES FOOD GET A FREE RIDE?

There's a little-known international treaty called the Convention on International Civil Aviation (signed in 1944), whose purpose was to help the fledgling airline industry. Under this treaty, fuel for international travel and transport of goods, including food, is exempt from taxes (unlike the fuel used for trucks, cars, and buses). There's also currently no tax on fuel used by ocean freighters, which hides the true "cost" of our current movable feast.[13]

EXOTIC SUPERFRUITS:
WORTH THE COST AND CARBON?

Move over mangoes and guavas—there's a whole new batch of exotic fruits hitting the markets these days. Hailing from exotic locales around the globe, they come steeped in intriguing cultural lore (some are said to improve your sex life) as well as 21st-century health claims (boosting immunity and fighting cancer). The question is, Are these superfruits worth it?

The bottom line: no. While they may add a splash of new taste or texture, or just make your diet seem more exotic, these fruits aren't any more likely to salve your American stress or provide a unique health advantage, and are likely to be a lot more carbon intensive. You will also likely pay more for them. So ignore the marketing hype (many of the claims are unsubstantiated) and save your dollars. Some fantastic American fruits that pack amazing nutrition include cranberries, pomegranates, blueberries, raspberries, blackberries, red grapes, and cherries.

Here's a quick rundown, with some suggestions of fantastic American beauties that may be a better bet when it comes to your health.[14]

FRUIT/LOCATION	FOUND IN	CLAIMS	AMERICAN BEAUTIES
Acai berry/Amazon	Juices and smoothies	Rich in anthocyanins, fiber, potassium, and magnesium	Blueberries or pomegranates
Goji berry/China	Juices and teas, breakfast cereals	High in beta-carotene, zeaxanthin, and lycopene	Tomatoes or dark, leafy greens
Noni/Tropics/ Southeast Asia	Juice, especially varieties sold online	Rich in vitamin C and potassium	Strawberries or raspberries
Mangosteen/ Africa, Asia, Pacific Tropics	Juices and desserts	Phytonutrients are extracted from its skin	Cranberries, red grapes, or cherries

Then there is a more practical consideration for those living in places where developers forgot to check with Mother Nature before plopping down communities; there may not actually *be* much local food. At least not all the time, anyway. Places like Arizona (the place, it's worth noting, from which Barbara Kingsolver fled in her best-selling *Animal, Vegetable, Miracle* in order to be able to get closer to her food), Nevada, and Utah come to mind, where much of the land is basically a desert. People in places such as Montana and Alaska contend with very short growing seasons. Is localism a sort of eco-fantasy for these folks? For some months of the year, probably yes.

So with all of these vagaries of the food system spelled out, you may be scratching your head at this point and asking yourself, "If it's not always greener, why should I bother to become a locavore?"

The answer is relatively simple: because many times, it *is* the greenest choice. And with spiraling energy prices, it is time to invest in the future of green local food. Now. What's more, eating more like a locavore makes for a smart strategy when it comes to getting lean.

THE HIGH COST OF CONVENIENCE

Simple is really a better deal for you and the planet in every way. Take a look at the premium you pay for "convenience," probably without knowing it.

FOOD ITEM	PRICE*	COST PER OUNCE
32-oz bag carrots	$1.79	5¢
10-oz bag shredded carrots	$1.49	14¢
Head romaine lettuce (36 oz)	$1.69	5¢
9-oz bag Fresh Express Chopped Romaine	$2.99	33¢
Musselman's Applesauce (48-oz jar)	$3.79	8¢
Six (4-oz) packs Musselman's Applesauce (24 oz total)	$2.99	12¢
Orville Redenbacher's Movie Theater Butter Gourmet Popping Corn (three 3-oz bags)	$2.99	30¢
Jolly Time Popcorn in resealable bag (32 oz)	$1.79	6¢

Prices from Albertsons Supermarket in Park City, Utah, on June 11, 2008.

AMERICA'S SHIFT FROM FOOD TO FOOD PRODUCTS:
HIGHER CALORIES, COST, AND CARBON PER SERVING[15]

FOOD	COST PER UNIT*	INDUSTRIAL "FOOD PRODUCTS"	COST PER UNIT*
Fresh ear of corn (90 calories)	60¢/ear	Cheese popcorn (160 calories per serving)	$1.79/bag (5 oz) 36¢/oz
		Corn chips (140 calories per serving)	$3.79/bag (13 oz) 29¢/oz
		Cornflakes (110 calories per serving)	$2.79/box (12 oz) 23¢/oz
Potato (130 calories)	70¢/lb 4¢/oz	Potato Au Gratin from a box (180 calories per 1-cup serving)	33¢/oz
		BBQ potato chips (150 calories per serving)	$3.79/bag 34¢/oz
		Frozen tater tots (170 calories per 9 tots)	$3.00/bag (2 lbs) 9¢/oz
Oatmeal (155 calories per serving)	$2.99/container (18 oz) 16¢/oz	Oatmeal bar (180 calories)	$3.39/box (6) 38¢/oz
Skinless, boneless chicken breasts (122 calories per 4-oz serving)	$4.29/lb 26¢/oz	Chicken nuggets (356 calories per 4-oz serving)	$4.99/package 41¢/oz
Fresh bacon (130 calories per 1-oz serving)	$3.49/8 oz 43¢/oz	Bacon bits (48 calories per 2 Tbsp)	$2.29/jar 76¢/oz

*Prices from Shaw's Supermarket, 71 Dodge Street, Beverly, MA 01915, on June 16, 2008.

Localism as a Lean Strategy

Perhaps one of the most important benefits to a more localized diet is that it's our best shot at reversing a disturbing trend nutritionists and dietitians around the country are seeing—many of us really don't *have* a relationship to food anymore.

People seem willing to put up with the tasteless offerings in the supermarket because they are steadily losing direct experience with what food actually tastes like. The dramatic flavor of a freshly picked raspberry, still warm from the sun, can stop you in your tracks. Do you remember your first experience where the power of flavor and taste did that?

I do. It was summertime, and I was in Pittsfield, Massachusetts, living with my grandmother while working at Tanglewood and writing my master's thesis. Having grown up in a house where we "made" salad for dinner from a box called "E tu Brute" (with a little picture of a laurelled Julius Caesar staring back from a box containing little pouches of croutons, "bacon" bits, Parmesan "cheese," and dressing), I equated food from a garden with my *Little House on the Prairie* phase when I was a tween.

Over for dinner at the home of family friends Gary and Carol Scarafoni, I wandered over to their garden more out of curiosity than any burning desire to know my food. But it was a revelation. I gobbled sugar snap peas still hanging on the vine. They were bursting with sweetness and crunch. They were alive. I never even knew I *liked* sugar snap peas—and I realized at that moment it was because I had never actually tasted them. I was suddenly *excited* to think about eating more of this stuff, because it tasted so much better! What else, I wondered, had I been missing out on all of these years? And why the heck were we eating salad from a *box* if things like this were out there?

Then, there's the added culinary advantage to eating like a locavore. "When you start with the best ingredients, you really don't need to do a lot to them because they will stand deliciously on their own," says Amanda Archibald, RD. Amanda's company, www.fieldtoplate.com, has one of the best seasonal resource guides available online; you can click on your state and get a customized guide of what is in season for that state each month during the year.

Iverson Brownell, owner of Iverson Catering in Park City, agrees. "Don't be intimidated by the idea of breaking out of your comfort zone when it comes to moving to seasonal produce," Brownell suggests. "The key is to try the same produce and cook it a few different ways to figure out what works best for your family. So, for instance, one day in spring, you may buy fresh asparagus and toss it on the grill with some olive oil, salt, and pepper; the next week, you may try roasting it in the oven at 375°F with the same dressing, but perhaps throw a bit of Parmesan cheese on it. Then the following week,

JOIN A CSA

The CSA (Community Supported Agriculture) concept originated in Japan 30 years ago. Called *teikei,* this translates to "putting the farmers' faces on food." Today there are more than 1,000 CSAs across the United States and Canada, and the number continues to expand.

Community Supported Agriculture lets you buy directly from the people who are growing your food, often allowing you to save money in the process. Farms typically invite members to buy a weekly "share" of food produced during the growing season.

Log on to www.localharvest.org to find the CSA or farmers' market nearest to you.

you cook it in a pan with the same dressing and give a nice squeeze of lemon juice at the end. After a few trials, you'll have a good idea of how you like to prepare your veggies, and what works specifically for your lifestyle and taste."

If local food tastes better, it's no surprise to learn that eating more like a locavore is a leaner bet. All things being equal, local food offers a higher-quality package than something shipped from miles away—often with less packaging. It slashes all that transit and storage time, keeping nutrients and phytochemicals intact. It will connect you more directly to those vibrant, fresh, living foods that create a greater vibrancy in your own body. It will force you to follow a more diverse diet that is a hallmark of healthier eating. And perhaps as an added bonus, it helps leverage your natural biology; you are apt to simply eat less if you don't have the world at your fingertips every time you get the slightest desire for a nibble. Of course, I am not suggesting we revert to our puritanical days, scrounging by on meager produce in winter, but clearly we need to strike a better balance. Localism can help. So while localism isn't a silver bullet for a diet to help stop global warming, it's still a very good strategy for other reasons. If you can't practice it all the time, *practice it as much as you can, to the extent that you can.*

A FRESH LOOK AT THE POWER OF PRODUCE

If farmers had the marketing muscle of pharmaceutical companies, we'd all be flocking to the produce aisle and duking it out over the last pint of blueberries. Here's a quick rundown of just some of the life-supporting benefits that research suggests fruits and vegetables have to offer. They:

- Contain compounds that help prevent and slow abnormal cell and tumor development, and encourage cell death in cancer cells

- Boost your memory and even reverse aging in the brain

- Stimulate your body to produce more natural killer cells to fight infection

- Act as natural antiviral and antifungal agents in the body

- Relax artery walls, fight clot formation, and reduce blood pressure levels

- Prevent your body from absorbing some of the cholesterol from the foods you eat

- Preserve lean muscle tissue

- Fight inflammation throughout many of your body's systems

- Alleviate arthritis and joint pain

- Act as a natural detox for harmful carcinogens

- Preserve your vision and protect your eyes from UV damage

- Keep skin, nails, and hair glowing

The best way to get excited about food is to bring it alive to your senses. Local food tastes better, and it's a powerful tool to get you to eat more healthfully. Many kids today have no connection to the food supply other than supermarket-sterile food sold in shiny wrappers, accompanied by lots of marketing, with no whiff of the farm or the animals that created it. Is this where food "comes from"? So teach your children well; instead of popping in a Baby Einstein DVD for them to learn about life on "Old MacDonald's farm" (which many of us have been guilty of, myself included), why not connect them in real life to the flavors of local food and the dynamics of the growing process? If you do, they are likely to get excited and actually *eat*. No matter where you live, from urban to rural, you can nourish those connections and plant the seeds of food for a lifetime. Research shows this not only boosts the odds that they will try some of those foods (which means better nutrition and eating habits), but you'll also be giving them valuable face time with Mother Earth, who desperately needs that generation to care.

TAKE ACTION NOW

- Ask your local market to start carrying more local produce options. Even if they can do it only in the summer months, it's an easy way to green up your cart and freshen the flavor (plus no additional trekking to the farmers' market).

- Join a local CSA to ensure that a portion of your produce is grown locally. Visit www.localharvest.org to find the CSA or farmers' market nearest you.

- Log on to www.fieldtoplate.com, click on "Resources," and download a copy of your own state's Seasonal Look Up Guide. Tape it to a door in your kitchen or somewhere in your pantry and get to know the seasons in your area.

- Check out the seasonal menus starting on page 228 and pick the lean and green eating plan that is in season right now.

- Log on to Harvest Eating (www.harvesteating.com) for super-easy and delicious recipes to help you make the leap from farm to table. You can download seasonal recipes, see what's growing in your area right now, and watch videos to brush up on your culinary skills.

- Keep your notions of "localism" less than puritanical. People in some parts of America can do it easily in 50 to 100 miles, while others may need to loosen that to 200 or so. Look within your town, then your state, then even your general region to scout out produce options.

So is it really so bad for the planet for you to be nibbling straw-berries in wintertime? Once in a while, probably not. But the inconvenient truth is that when it is a standard part of 300 million Americans' diets, alongside a pile of other utterly unsustainable choices, yes.

In the end, it's really pretty simple.

Eat fresh, vibrant, seasonal food. As much as you can.

A win for you. A win for the planet.

EASY, IMMEDIATE SAVINGS: SHOP EFFICIENTLY

Here's another immediate, easy way that you can inch into a greener zone: Even if you don't change what's in your cart, if you simply reduce how often you fill it, you can take a big bite out of your carbon footprint. That's because your ride as a personal shopper is probably going to be the *least* efficient leg of your food's journey. In fact, a professor at UC Davis determined that, for the same amount of fuel, 11 pounds of groceries would travel:

1 kilometer by private car

43 kilometers by air

740 kilometers by truck

2,400 kilometers by rail

3,800 kilometers by ship[16]

What's the take-home point for you?

For one thing, zipping to the farmers' market in your SUV for organic strawberries is *not* greener for the Earth. With more than half of all Americans living in suburbia (requiring a car trip for all errands), savings matter.

So identify at least two ways you can personally become a more efficient shopper. Can you shop less frequently? Bring your own bags? Get a carpool going to the big box retailer with some neighbors or send your list of requests to a friend and take turns going? Split up mega orders for cost and carbon savings? Remember that your personal food miles are as much a factor in a greener diet as almost anything else.

PORTION SIZES
=
PANTS SIZE

Welcome to Part IV of your program. Here in week 5, your goal is to bring the portion sizes of some of your most bloated food items back into a better balance for vitality, health, weight, and carbon footprint.

Part IV also tackles one of the biggest elephants in the room, industrial food. We're eating less "food" today and more "food products." We rise and shine with "food" that seems more appropriate for someone on the NASA space station rather than a child heading off to school—highly processed, shrink-wrapped in enough packaging to survive the next Katrina, specifically engineered to overwhelm the senses with salty, sweet, or one of a zillion flavors, and containing a smattering of nutrients tossed in to fool us into thinking it's "healthy." It's confusing, it's overwhelming, and too much of it is unhealthy for your body and for the planet.

It's time to redefine the idea of a "value meal" with one that doesn't cost more, or take any more time to make. While each chapter delves into great detail, here is the "Cliffs Notes" version, as well as the specific action steps you can take *now*.

GET STARTED NOW: REAL, SIMPLE SOLUTIONS TO START LOSING TODAY

1 REDISCOVER ANCIENT GRAINS. Packed with nutrition, health benefits, and slimming power, ancient grains are making a comeback to a supermarket near you. It's time to start eating more of these delicious grains, in the right amounts to feel full and satisfied while also taking a bite out of your carbon.

2 CUT THE CRAP. Cut back on highly refined, highly processed, and packaged food products. You'll slow your carbon burn and possibly blood sugar swings (which can cause cravings).

3 FOCUS ON LEAN, CLEAN FATS. Purge the super-high-carbon trans fats from your pantry, and focus on fats that move you to better health and weight instead.

CHAPTER 10

GREAT GRAINS FOR A GREENER LIFESTYLE

"The whole argument that living a sustainable life is just for the élite isn't true. There are things . . . that are within the grasp of all of us."

—Michael Oshman, founder, Green Restaurant Association

YOUR LEAN AND GREEN PRESCRIPTION

5 to 6 servings per day of all-natural whole grains, as unrefined as possible

Serving size: ½ cup cooked grain, 1 ounce cereal,* 1 slice bread**

*Look for cereals with a minimum of 4 grams of fiber per serving and no more than 5 grams of sugar per serving; **Whole grain should be the first ingredient (minimum of 2 grams of fiber per slice)

INCLUDE

Whole grains (such as millet, oatmeal, amaranth, barley, bulgur, buckwheat, couscous, quinoa, spelt, polenta, wheat berries, and kasha)

Semolina or whole wheat pasta; buckwheat or soba noodles

Breads, crackers, pitas, naan, English muffins, lavash, rolls, and wraps made with whole grain flours (including whole wheat pastry flour)

Brown or wild rice as well as wheat or oat bran

All-natural whole grain pancake or waffle mix (or whole grain frozen waffles)

Naked popcorn kernels (popped with a small amount of clean fat)

Greenest: Minimal packaging (bulk is best), local products (i.e., local breads or granolas), no trans fats or partially hydrogenated oils, organic

AVOID

Refined breads, cereals, and grain products and white "whole grain" products (including those listing "wheat flour" or "flour")

High-fat breads such as croissants, biscuits, scones, pastries, toaster pastries, and doughnuts; high-fat, buttery crackers

Sugary or refined-grain breakfast cereals, pancakes, or waffles

Energy, breakfast, and snack bars (unless they are whole grain and have a clean ingredient list, and you can afford the calories)

Single-serving or highly packaged grain products (e.g., 100-calorie snack packs) without clean ingredient lists

Now that you've already done a great job tackling legumes and dairy products, we'll spend week 5 cleaning up your grains to be greener, healthier, and more sustainable in every sense. By the end of this chapter, you'll see just how easy it is to serve up grains that leave you feeling satisfied and energized, and you'll clear the clutter from your pantry, your life, and your backside. You'll continue your journey to lighter living, in every sense of the word. It's not as tall an order as it may seem.

So let's start with a quick discussion of all that is to be gained from the grains in your Lean and Green Prescription.

LEAN BENEFITS

The lean and green overlap here is simple. More than 20 percent of the carbohydrates in the average American diet come from high-carbon, high-calorie foods, including soft drinks and soda (10 percent), cakes, cookies, quick breads, and doughnuts (7 percent), and sugars, syrups, and jams (6 percent).[1] Minimize those inputs and you'll automatically reap big savings in carbon *and* calories.

You see, just as not all fats are created equal, neither are carbohydrates. Unlike the refined carbohydrates mentioned in the high-carbon examples above, whole grains are a key part of a delicious and healthy low-carbon lifestyle. These "greener grains" are rich in the healthy kinds of carbohydrates that keep you feeling fuller longer and fight a slew of diseases, including heart disease, stroke, diverticulosis, insulin sensitivity, metabolic syndrome, and diabetes, all in a modest calorie package.

In addition to those benefits, there may be an added "lean factor" targeting another scourge, that tough-to-lose belly fat; some research suggests a calorie-controlled diet rich in whole grains may play a role in helping to shed belly fat. A 2008 study in the *American Journal of Clinical Nutrition,* for example, tracked two groups following similar lower-calorie diets and found that while both lost weight, the group that ate whole grains shed significantly more belly fat and slashed the levels of inflammatory proteins in their blood by 38 percent, a level of decrease similar to that attained by using *statin drugs.*[2] Like I said, Mother Nature's pharmacy in action.

Plus, because unrefined whole grains come in the natural package that nature intended, they provide more trace minerals, fiber, phytochemicals, and even healthy fats. They take longer to digest, so they fight hunger longer, and they keep your blood sugar stable longer. Their richer textures and flavors add a delicious, deeper element to food. And perhaps best of all, this is a relatively easy swap for most of my clients because these "green grains" still resemble many of the comfort foods we love; you can enjoy them as hearty side dishes and in casseroles, pancakes, and even the occasional cookie and muffin.

Because it's so important to savor whole grains in the right amounts, you'll need to keep two things in mind. Number one, all grains are *not* created equal; stick as much as you can to minimally processed whole grains and ancient grains, and limit or avoid refined grains (such as white flour) and food products that feature them. These types of foods can cause high glycemic loads, which then spike blood sugar, triglyceride levels, and insulin levels, and have been shown to trigger inflammation and lower "good" HDL cholesterol.

The second key is *moderation.* If you plow through piles of refined grains, pastas, and dinner rolls regularly, you will fatten up as quickly as those cows doing the same thing in the feedlot that you've just left behind.

Let's take pasta, for example, which many of my clients instantly tag as "fattening"—something to be avoided alongside candy bars and soda. Having lived in Italy for 2 years, I can tell you with certainty that the portions of pasta they're serving up in Florence and Rome bear no resemblance whatsoever to the mega portions of pasta heaped onto plates at your typical Italian chain restaurant here in America. Across the pond, diners get an average of 1½ to 2 cups of pasta in total (3 to 4 servings). Those on *this* side of the Atlantic, in contrast, can pack a whopping 5 to 8 cups (10 to 16 servings) on a plate at a time! This gives us a small window into why our butts are bigger on this side of the Atlantic as well.

SIZING UP YOUR SERVINGS

Size matters. Big time. Your portion sizes are directly linked to your pants size, so let's define a couple of things.

"Portion" is a loose measurement. It simply refers to the amount of food you eat at a given time. You could as easily say "a plate of pasta," a "bowl of ice cream," or "a bottle of soda." All are vague.

A "serving," in contrast, is a specific amount of food with a defined nutrient range. Servings are expressed in units of measurement, such as cups, teaspoons, or ounces.

Therefore, a "portion" of food on your plate can often amount to several servings. If you're trying to slim down, it's obviously key to keep portions within your calorie needs. That's why the Go Green Get Lean Diet gives you specific serving guidelines (i.e., ounces or cups) within each food group, all designed to keep you on around a 1,600-calorie diet.

In my opinion, the real value of "serving sizes" is to retrain your eyes as to how much food is appropriate for your plate. In our supersized world, most of us have lost this skill. Often, after a couple of weeks of closely watching servings, you will learn how to "eyeball it," thereby freeing up time in the kitchen. But if you're watching your weight or trying to lose, I strongly suggest you measure things out about once a week to make sure you're looking with "honest eyeballs," as one client calls it. Here are a few guidelines for what these servings look like:

A SERVING OF THIS FOOD	LOOKS LIKE THIS
A medium piece of fruit	A baseball (if you're a woman, the size of your fist)
½ cup of whole grains or pasta	Computer mouse
3 ounces of meat, poultry, or fish	A deck of cards or a checkbook
1 ounce of cheese	Four dice or two dominoes
1 tablespoon of peanut butter or fat	The tip of your thumb or a postage stamp

Most experts will advise you to split an entrée. It's a great idea, but in our supersized culture, even that doesn't really go far enough anymore. It's definitely a start, but the problem is that while we know it's a *big* plate, most of us have no idea just how big. And unless we bother to actually measure the exact item (which most of us, myself included, usually don't), we have no way of knowing.

So know this: Often, even if you split these mega portions with a friend, you've still blown through your entire grain budget in one sitting. So bone up on serving sizes as a good defense against "grain bloat."

Other carb pitfalls to watch for include bagels large enough to feed a small village; jumbo "muffins" (which are usually, let's be frank, cake sold at breakfast time) that pack the caloric heft of a stick of butter, and almost as much saturated fat; and that tub of buttery popcorn at the movie theater large enough to lose your first-born child in (that for some reason is priced cheaper than the smallest box). Others? Focaccia breads and "panini" sandwiches that pack a day's worth of grains in a single sitting. Your local pancake house that promises your pic on the wall and a free breakfast if you can finish their "jumbo stack" of pancakes in under an hour. In American culture, the list goes on and on.

The right kinds, in the right amounts. Say it with me. When it comes to grains, this is your road map for lighter, leaner living.

So let's talk about green cuisine that gets you lean, shall we?

GREEN BENEFITS

Now that you're a flexitarian, you're already greener with your grains, and here's why: About 70 percent of all grain production in the United States goes toward feeding livestock. Hence, it's much, much more energy efficient to eliminate the middleman (or middle cow, so to speak).

Though there isn't currently information available to the consumer on the specific carbon footprint of one type of grain over another, we can still use the guideposts that we *do* have about food in general to make better choices. I like to think of these guideposts as the Three Cs: Carbon, Calories, and Cost. Factors that raise carbon (and often calories and cost) include:

- The amount of processing and packaging required
- The length and contents of the ingredient list

THE FIBER FACTOR:
START LOOKING AND FEELING FABULOUS

Personally, I think fiber's reputation could use a makeover. Just as "dried California plums" sounds a whole lot more exciting and delicious than "prunes," to most people, fiber is long overdue for a publicist. But don't let that stop you from loving fiber. Moving back to whole grains and experimenting with the "newer" ancient grains that are making a comeback will help you easily meet your goals.

Aim for about 30 grams of fiber a day (most Americans get about half that). Fiber plays an essential role in keeping you trim and healthy. Here's how:

■ Fiber helps with elimination, keeping belly bloating in check.

■ Fiber helps buffer insulin and blood sugar swings, taming cravings.

■ Fiber keeps you fuller longer by slowing transit time from the stomach, which is key to effectively eating less without being hungry.

■ Fiber helps lower "bad" LDL cholesterol levels, keeping your heart healthy.

■ High-fiber foods take longer to chew and eat, giving your brain time to catch up with your stomach when you sense you're full; it's very easy to blow through that window when you're eating highly refined, high-calorie, already-prepared, easy-to-access food such as fast food and snack food products.

■ High-fiber diets give you more volume with fewer calories—a key secret to lasting weight loss.

■ The temperature gauge (Frozen? Chilled? Needing to be reheated? Or is it shelf stable and can be eaten that way?)
■ Whether it's organic or conventional, local or global
■ How much development/marketing/advertising is behind the product

To illustrate the Three Cs in action, one research study calculated that a 2-pound box of breakfast cereal requires about four times as many fossil fuel calories to produce as is actually in the cereal itself, burning about a half gallon of gasoline.[3] This doesn't include the carbon included in marketing, transportation, or your personal trip to the store in your car. While such a number isn't useful in a vacuum (Is it better or worse than, say, crackers, chips, or a fruit roll-up, or that organic quinoa in bulk?), it is helpful to highlight the carbon-intense nature of processed food. Consider that if only *half* of all Americans ate one of these boxes of cereal a month, over a year the production alone would require 900 million gallons of gasoline. One food choice.

One of perhaps dozens you make every day.

If you stick to whole grains that are minimally processed, minimize excessive packaging, choose easy-to-read ingredient lists, and put your food dollars in companies with strong sustainability initiatives, you'll be taking four steps to cool your carbon. If you can go organic, that's great—go ahead and buy those organic crackers. It certainly may be an added plus; you'll be saving the fossil fuel that comes with all of those pesticides and fertilizers. However, I personally recommend that if you have a limited budget for organics, it is probably more important to buy organic animal products and produce first. The health trade-offs are worth it.

TAKE ACTION NOW

Out with the old. Check out the labels on your cereals, crackers, rice, snacks, grain side dishes, and breads. Make sure they make the nutrition cut; they should be whole grain with absolute minimal amounts of white flour, refined sugars, refined grains, and ingredients that require a PhD in chemical speak. Next, check the fiber content. Ideally, clear out and donate anything that isn't moving you toward leaner and greener living. Alternately, "flag" those items that you'll not buy again (with a black marker, a Post-it note, or whatever works for you), and start scanning the market on your next trip for a suitable swap. (You can also print out a copy of your lean and green shopping list at www.leanandgreendiet.com to bring with you to the store.)

In with the new. For a fun change of pace in your kitchen, build a pantry that combines the power of healthy foods with the power of

YOUR L.E.A.N. CHEAT SHEET

So many questions go into making the greenest choices, and the irony is that there's a lot of micro information (Does this company use wind power? Is there LED lighting in that production plant? What's the mileage efficiency of the fleet of trucks they use?) that is nearly impossible to obtain. And I'm here to say *that is okay.* You'll get paralyzed into inaction if you seek every single detail (which, frankly, is changing daily anyway as companies try to green up their acts).

So instead, try your hand with this handy acronym to see if something is truly L.E.A.N. in that it's good for both your waistline and the planet. You can use it anywhere, anytime you're about to put something into your mouth.

Local or global?

Energy used to bring it to your plate? (Include processing, packaging, transportation, and temperature of food.)

Animal or plant? (Plant foods are greener.)

Necessary? (Is it critical to meet your health and weight goals?)

What you will usually find when you use this method is that it consistently brings you to a place that, if not the perfect shade of green (because researchers would have to specifically do a custom carbon count for your personal scenario), is certainly pretty close. Of course, there are always going to be some exceptions (such as fish), and there are still vigorous debates around the very methods being used to determine carbon footprint. So don't worry about getting bogged down in the minutiae; leave that to the energy experts who are meticulously teasing out each strand in the global warming ball.

Besides, getting bogged down makes it easy to miss the bigger point; your goal is to trim your waistline and your carbon footprint—to *look* great while you *do* great by the Earth. Being a point off here or there is small potatoes compared with the biggest pieces of your diet: Invest your energy in focusing on other areas of your diet where environmental and health implications are more significant. Where you eat on the food chain. The amount you waste. Your shopping habits. These, at the end of the day, are likely to cut your carbon a lot more than switching to organic crackers.

good taste. Hit the market (load up from the bulk bins to curb your carbon even more) and welcome the following new pals to lean and green living, including some ancient grains that are making a comeback. Put them in old glass jam jars or another "reusable," and you've shed even more carbon and will have a pantry that would make Martha Stewart proud.

Old-fashioned oatmeal: One of the original health foods. Skip the sugary packets and go back to the lower-carbon original. It cooks in about 5 minutes. If you like, mix it with another multigrain breakfast cereal to shake things up a bit.

Breakfast cereal in bags, not boxes: Buy cereal that's in one layer of plastic packaging rather than in boxes (which have cardboard *and* plastic packaging) for immediate carbon savings. These "eco-pacs" can save up to 60 percent of packaging over regular boxes, and often save you money as well; Nature's Path, for instance, now puts their healthy, yummy, whole grain cereals in eco-pacs that are much greener for the Earth and a better bet for your wallet, too.

Quinoa: Originating in South America, quinoa is loaded with high-quality protein and iron. It is as versatile as rice, has a mild nutty flavor, and is delicious as a hot breakfast cereal, a stuffing in vegetables, or a chilled salad.

Bulgur: A high-fiber grain popular in Middle Eastern dishes such as tabbouleh, bulgur cooks quickly and makes an amazing hot or cold dish when tossed with nuts, dried fruit, herbs, and beans.

Barley: Chewy and meaty, barley has a slow digestive time that keeps hunger at bay and insulin levels stable for hours. It's awesome for hearty winter soups (especially when paired with mushrooms).

Wheat berries: If you're feeling adventurous, wheat berries pack amazing nutrition and a dense, nutty flavor. And the taste just gets better the longer it sits, making tasty leftovers a snap.

Boxed grains: Easy peasy time-savers. There are several great shortcut products being made by companies with an eye toward a healthy body and Earth. Bob's Red Mill is a fave (and a great source of high-quality gluten-free products). As an added plus, they come in minimal packaging and contain nothin' but clean ingredients. Seeds of Change and Kashi also both have some amazing "heat and go" whole grains. Just zap and serve. (To keep an eye on salt, I suggest you use only half the seasoning pack. You can use the rest to season some bulk grains at another meal.) Yes, these products are a bit higher carbon than hitting the bulk bin, but they're still a great way to ease your toe into green cuisine if you lack culinary confidence or need to strike a balance with a time-strapped reality.

Better bread: It's getting easier and easier to find delicious, clean, even artisan bread at supermarkets across the country as demand has zoomed and people are beginning to realize that the squishy white stuff with a 6-year expiration date just isn't that tasty. Ideally, the ingredient list on your bread will read pretty close to: "flour, water, yeast, salt." Choose one layer of packaging instead of two, and cut packaging by 20 percent for each gram of bread.

Create a "locals only" shelf. Whether they're grain products or not, choose two or three food items that you use a lot and begin to source them locally, if you can, or even regionally. Create a space in both your pantry and your fridge for the locals. Keeping a separate space will help you see how much in your diet is local. For instance, here in Utah we have a great tortilla chip company, raw honey, an all-natural salsa/guacamole company, a raw milk cheese producer, a local coffee roaster, and even a local energy bar. While localism isn't a catchall answer to the carbon crisis, it is certainly *part* of the solution and has many other healthy benefits as well.

Dine out—deliciously. When eating out, order brown rice instead of white, ask for a pizza made with a whole wheat crust, or order whole wheat pasta. Try the new vegetarian or vegan restaurant in town (there are more every year). Their menus can help you ease into these new exotic grains, and they often feature amazing flavors that highlight cuisine from around the globe.

In the next chapter, we're moving on to tackle one of the biggest elephants in the room when it comes to your diet: dietary fats. Are you ready? Good. Here comes the fun part.

It's time to lighten the junk in your trunk.

CHAPTER 11

FATS: THE LEAN, THE GREEN, AND THE MEAN

"Believe you can or believe you can't. Either way you will be right.**"**

—Henry Ford

YOUR LEAN AND GREEN PRESCRIPTION
up to 6 teaspoons per day

INCLUDE DAILY

Monounsaturated fats (preferably unrefined, cold pressed if oils)

Omega-3 fats

(Note: For each serving of your higher-fat, healthy, whole foods, such as nuts, seeds, avocados, and olives, simply count 1 of your fat teaspoons toward each serving.)

Greener: Organic, sold in a larger container or bulk (minimize packaging). For oils, choose cold expeller pressed or extra virgin. Local if possible.

LIMIT (INCLUDE MONTHLY)

Omega-6 fats (unrefined and cold pressed)

Saturated fat from butter—preferably local, organic, grass fed. (When you do use butter, which should be sparingly, make sure it's good quality.)

AVOID

Trans fats, partially hydrogenated oils

Margarines and shortenings. (One possible exception is if you have high cholesterol and are using a plant sterol–based spread as part of an overall diet strategy.)

Lard

Saturated fats in beef, dairy, and other animal products. (Stick to your other Lean and Green Prescription amounts.)

Here's a fact that may surprise you: The *total* amount of fat you eat (whether high or low) isn't really linked with disease. Rather, it's the *type* of fat you eat that matters most. Here's another interesting fact: Eating enough fat is one of the secrets of being able to stick with a healthier diet for the long haul.

The right kinds, in the right amounts. Once again.

If the new green cuisine is about healthy and fresh foods, cooked in healthy and fresh ways, fat is one of the central players in this new lifestyle. Why? Fat adds flavor, mouth appeal, and texture to foods, which is why we love it so much (and why many of us didn't feel satisfied when we followed the fat-free craze). It also does something deeper: Fat provides staying power to foods because it takes longer to digest than carbohydrate. This means that you will be fuller longer if you include some fat in your meals and snacks.

Here's more good news: If you've been following each part of your program thus far, including your Lean and Green Prescriptions and "Take Action Now" steps, you have already done a fantastic job realigning nearly all of your fats to be cleaner, healthier, and in better amounts. Specifically, you're a flexitarian, including fish, wild game, and nuts and more plant proteins in your diet; you are a sustainable snacker; and you're cooking more of your food at home. All of these changes help you mount your best defense against the typical Western eating pattern, which is too high in saturated fat, trans fats, and even omega-6 fats, and sets us up for many of our leading diseases and low-grade systemic inflammation. Good for you.

During the next phase of your pantry purge, you'll complete your transformation by stocking up on antiaging, anti-inflammatory, beautylicious fats and eliminating the remaining aging, artery-clogging, high-carbon ones for good. Time to separate the clean and green from the mean.

LEAN BENEFITS

I'll admit, fats are complicated. For one, many people find the idea of eating the right fats in order to lose body fat confusing. Then there are all the nuances among the different types: Which are good? Which are bad? And how much of each should be included in a healthy diet? For some reason, even my own mother, who has no trouble at all remembering that "wine is great for you," is still wary of peanut butter, nuts, and avocados because they're "loaded with fat." I have to constantly remind her that these good fats will help her look fabulous well into her sixties, and they may even keep her off of the medication that so many people her age are on. But I can understand her confusion.

So, keeping Mom (and everyone like her) in mind, I've done the work for you to keep things simple. If you like, simply look at the table on page 161 for your list of "lean and clean" fats to include, stick to your Prescription amounts, and you're off and running. If you want to learn the "why" behind it, or brush up on your fat facts, read on.

Your Prescription is designed to realign your fats in the following ways.

1. **Emphasize the lean and clean fats.** All of your Prescriptions work together to enhance your diet with the right kinds of fats.

2. **Bring a better balance.** While we do need some omega-6 fats in our diets, we need smaller amounts than most of us are getting. Further, it's critical that they are the highest quality—unrefined and cold pressed as opposed to highly processed. Your Prescription rebalances your ratio of omega-3 to omega-6 fats in a way that promotes maximum health and minimizes inflammation.

3. **Eliminate the worst offenders.** You will purge your diet of the highest-carbon fats that are also terrible for your health.

4. **Get you to the right amounts.** You'll strike that winning balance between taste, health, and a healthy body weight.

So how does fat get you lean? Research suggests that eating heart-healthy fats actually helps with weight loss and assists in regulating body weight, all while fighting type 2 diabetes in the process.[1] So reserving a portion of your calories for these types of fats is a winning strategy.

But while research in a calorie-controlled food lab is great, how it translates to *your* own dinner table is what matters. So here's the added plus: Including heart-healthy fats in your diet is simply tasty and appealing to stick with.

One of the reasons the Mediterranean style of eating has become such a popular icon for weight loss and health is because it's delicious in the process. While there are other equally effective roads to better health and weight (the Dean Ornish or the Okinowan plans are two wonderful examples), in my experience these plans might be a bit too restrictive for many people to find lasting pleasure and lasting success when following them as a style of eating. The Go Green Get Lean Diet isn't an exact Mediterranean diet, but it leverages this same powerful truth: Fat sells.

So "know thyself"; and if thyself likes to enjoy higher-fat foods on occasion, it's critical to find a way to include them regularly. And because I know *myself,* I've designed the Go Green Get Lean Diet with that in mind. I've included just the right amount to help give you the most flavor, nutrition, and taste while keeping calories sustainable for your backside. If you're not concerned about weight loss, you can be more liberal with the amounts, but stick to the "clean and lean" categories for the maximum in clean and green overlap.

Of course, as I've already stressed, if you are trying to slim down, portions are important. And while you don't need a tight fist with veggies, fruits, and beans, fat is in a league of its own. That's because fat is the most energy-dense nutrient, weighing in at 9 calories per gram, more than twice the calories of protein or carbohydrate. In fact, 1 tablespoon of fat packs about 100 to 120 calories.

While all fat has the same amount of calories per gram, the *type* of fat you eat has a deep impact on your health. Again, it's the package that matters. Think, for a moment, about why your mother always told you to pour bacon grease into a can and not down the drain—because you don't want it to clog the pipes in your home. The same thing holds true for your own *personal* pipes (your arteries) when you eat saturated and trans fats. And here's a little-known fact: Trans fats were originally created to be used in candle wax. Trans fat is great for industrial food because it extends the shelf life by hundreds of years, but it's horrible for your personal pipes.

To be sure, fat alone could fill its own book. But the table on the next page offers you a quick primer on the clean, the lean, and the mean.

FAT FACTS: SEPARATING THE CLEAN AND LEAN FROM THE MEAN

Simply put, monounsaturated and omega-3 fats are lean and clean because they help keep you satisfied and fuller longer, help control blood sugar swings, and may help you lose weight and keep it off.[2] They may also help keep your skin beautiful and glowing, act as an anti-inflammatory in the body, keep your arteries clean and healthy, reduce blood pressure, and give your "good" cholesterol a boost. And they might even boost your brainpower (60 percent of the brain's weight is made up of fat).

Your Prescription limits saturated fat significantly and eliminates dirty trans fats altogether. Too much of these fats acts as a pro-inflammatory in the body and can clog your arteries, raise your risk of heart disease, and accelerate the accumulation of abdominal fat that leads to an "apple shape."[3] Plus, they can sap your energy and may raise your risk of dementia and Alzheimer's.

MONO	OMEGA-3	OMEGA-6	SATURATED	TRANS
Oils: Canola oil Flaxseed oil Olive oil Peanut oil *Foods:* Almonds Avocados Flaxseed Olives Peanuts Macadamia nuts Dark chocolate	*Oils:* Canola oil Fish oil Flaxseed oil Walnut oil *Foods:* Fish (especially fatty fish, such as anchovies, herring, sardines, salmon, tuna, and mackerel) Walnuts Wild game	*Oils:* Corn oil Cottonseed oil Grapeseed oil Safflower oil Sesame oil Soybean oil* Sunflower oil* *Foods:* Poultry Wild game	*Fats/Oils:* Butter Coconut oil Cocoa butter Margarine Palm oil *Foods:* Dairy fat Lamb/mutton Pork fat Red meat Coconut	*Fats/Oils:* Partially hydrogenated oils Hydrogenated oils Margarine spreads** *Foods:* (varies: read labels) Fried foods Cookies, pastries, pies, and doughnuts Nondairy creamer Crackers Chips

*Contain both omega-3 and omega-6 fats, but the oils are listed in the category where the contribution is more significant.

**Depends on individual spread; read the label.

Another benefit to these healthy fats? When your food choices are lean and green, you're eating foods that can help calm inflammation. Quite literally, these foods can help you slow the clock.

Chronic, systemic low-grade inflammation is an underlying factor of nearly every degenerative disease, including obesity, heart disease, diabetes, insulin resistance, autoimmune disease, chronic fatigue, weight gain, food sensitivities, and metabolic syndrome. It's no wonder millions of Americans report "GI troubles" to their physicians each year. With two-thirds of your immune system residing in your gut, it's often one of the first places where signs of inflammation (bloating, diarrhea, etc.) can show up. Some evidence suggests that inflammation slows weight loss, promotes weight gain, and ages you more quickly. Here are a few tips for calming inflammation.

WHAT TO EAT TO AVOID INFLAMMATION

ANTI-INFLAMMATORY FOODS	PRO-INFLAMMATORY FOODS
Omega-3 fats Blueberries, cherries, pomegranates, red cabbage, and beets (These foods are all high in antioxidants, and especially in anthocyanins, which are nature's COX-2 inhibitors.) Green tea and ginger	Omega-6 fats Trans fats Many margarines Fried foods Refined carbohydrates (white flour, refined sugars) Alcohol in excess
ANTI-INFLAMMATORY BEHAVIORS	PRO-INFLAMMATORY BEHAVIORS
Not smoking Healthy, manageable stress levels Rest and sleep	Smoking High stress levels Lack of sleep

While we're on the subject of inflammation and dietary fat, let's talk for a minute about your own body fat. While most of us would like to feel fewer wibbly wobblies on our arms or backsides (and of course, exercise will help tighten that), *where* fat hangs out on your body makes a big difference to your health, too.

Your fat stores are more than just your own personal Department of Energy storing excess fuel for a rainy day. Fat is a metabolically active organ, receiving and sending signals to and from other organs in your body. And just like real estate, it's all about location, location, location.

Subcutaneous fat (the aforementioned wibbly wobbly bits) may be unpleasant to you, but it's relatively harmless compared to the fat that resides around your middle. Belly fat, located in your midsection and clinically known as more benign-sounding "visceral fat," lies in between your stomach muscles and vital organs. This is the fat that can give you an "apple shape" with a big belly, and it is directly linked to higher rates of diabetes, heart disease, and metabolic syndrome. It's also linked to higher rates of nasty inflammation in your body.

Belly fat is directly impacted by how sedentary you are. The more time in front of the TV or computer or being a couch potato, the more likely you are to carry a hefty middle. Good-bye skinny jeans, hello elastic waistband.

Fortunately, although it is a complicated element in many of our food choices, managing the amount of fat in your diet is a key part of living a leaner lifestyle. The table below illustrates how just a few easy swaps can trim calories—and carbon—from your diet.

SIX SIMPLE SWAPS TO LEANER, GREENER FUELS

INSTEAD OF THIS	CHOOSE THIS	SAVE THIS
Butter, 2 Tbsp on toast, 200 calories	Hummus, 2 Tbsp on toast, 50 calories	150 calories
Mayo, 2 Tbsp on sandwich, 200 calories	Grainy mustard, 2 Tbsp on sandwich, 20 calories	180 calories
1 cup chocolate premium ice cream 380 calories	1 cup 100 percent local fruit sorbet 266 calories	114 calories
1 slice Cheddar cheese on sandwich 110 calories	½ cup sprouts and ½ cup baby spinach on sandwich 5 calories	105 calories
16 oz pumpkin spice latte 380 calories	16 oz nonfat latte 130 calories	250 calories
2 cups microwave popcorn 130 calories	2 cups homemade popcorn cooked in canola oil 83 calories	47 calories

GREEN BENEFITS

Here's one way you probably haven't thought about that your new lean and green lifestyle is going to trim your carbon footprint—helping to reduce carbon dioxide emissions the next time you step on an airplane. Seems overpacked suitcases aren't the only thing weighing down the friendly skies these days. A 2004 Centers for Disease Control and Prevention (CDC) study found that because of the average 10-pound weight gain of Americans in the 1990s, in 2000 airlines burned an additional 350 million gallons of gasoline just to fly that extra poundage, releasing an extra 3.8 million tons of carbon dioxide into the atmosphere.[5]

Another hidden benefit? Significant fuel savings on the road—in fact, keeping your tires pumped up is small potatoes compared to the fuel savings of keeping your waistline slim. That's because every 1-pound increase in the average per-passenger weight in America translates to approximately 39.2 million gallons of extra gasoline that are required to transport that extra weight. In fact, experts estimate that nearly one billion additional gallons of fuel are burned annually in the United States each year to tote around all our extra pounds gained since the 1960s.[6] It seems fuel efficiency of cars may have less of an impact on greenhouse gas emissions than would stemming our obesity crisis. My goodness.

But back to fats. When it comes to looking at fats with an eye for green, let's use a hypothetical situation. Suppose the question is, "If you live closer to a dairy farm than an olive grove (which, let's be honest, most Americans do), does this give you the green light to slather on the butter instead of opting for that virginal olive oil?"

Nice try.

Eating clean fat is such a critical part of creating better health and making it easier to lose weight and keep it off, that this is one area where it seems wiser to strike a balance between health and carbon cost. While they may be local, animal fats still aren't green. So eat only as much as your Prescription allows, or perhaps a small bit more if your calorie intake is much higher.

For the small amounts of butter in your diet, yes, choose local to the extent that you can. Even better if it's grass fed or organic (and you may notice this butter has an amazing flavor, reflecting what the cows ate). But cows and cow products are still likely to be the SUVs of your diet—even a local cow.

As it is with fish, the exact carbon count of your fat is going to be hard to determine. Indeed, much olive oil in the United States is imported, which certainly flies in the face of localism. Yet clean fat is still in the plant kingdom, so might we be able to hedge our bets a bit and salve our conscience, thinking that plant foods are better? I think so. In addition, here are a few other reasons that make the carbon case for sticking to lean and clean.

- The worst offenders, the trans fats, are found primarily in high-carbon foods such as processed foods and convenience foods. Or they're coming from deep-fried food at a restaurant, which is also a higher-carbon (not to mention higher-calorie) eating situation.

- Most animal fats require extensive refrigeration (e.g., cheese, butter, sour cream, milk, yogurt, and ice cream), which creates additional carbon emissions during transport and storage. In contrast, most vegetable fats can safely be stored at room temperature. This is a much more carbon-friendly place in the 18-wheeler, the supermarket, and your pantry.

- Your clean and lean fats don't have to be globe-trotters. For those living in the western United States, California olive oil is a nice lean and green overlap. Canola oil and flax oil can be found closer to home. (Canola oil is actually a modified grapeseed oil, named "canola" oil by Canada.) Chances are good your canola oil comes from North America. Other items such as avocados, walnuts, olives, almonds, and local fish may also be closer to home.

- Even those living far away from an olive grove can take comfort in the fact that olive oil is shipped in energy-efficient ways (such as cargo ships from Europe), unlike produce, wine, and other sensitive items (which are often flown). So while not the deepest shade of green, it's likely not swimming in fossil fuels, either.

So stick to your Lean and Green Prescription even if you're smack-dab in the middle of dairy country. Even if you're off a carbon point or two, don't sweat it. Use Your L.E.A.N. Cheat Sheet (see page 154) to keep you pointed in the right direction. Green up your saturated fats by looking for local dairy products or meats, which will be fresher and help cut food miles. And be sure to eliminate the *mean*—those nasty trans fats. They are high carbon, aging, and pro-inflammatory; they may hasten that lovely "apple shape" of fat deposits; and they may harden your arteries. Why is that such a problem? Your arteries are your lifelines. Literally.

TAKE ACTION NOW

- **Enjoy olive oil and canola oil and don't sweat the food miles.** Choose extra virgin olive oil and cold expeller-pressed canola, peanut, or other oils. (Spectrum is a great brand that's available in most markets.) Store in a cool, dark place (not right near the stove) for maximum shelf life. I suggest starting with medium sizes (as opposed to super bulk) until you know how quickly you go through them. And make sure you recycle the containers.

- **Enjoy foods that pack clean fats.** These include avocados, olives, flaxseed, and nuts. (Store nuts in the freezer; see page 99 for a list of recommended nuts.)

- **Think locally when choosing dairy.** See the guidelines in Chapter 8 on page 108.

- **Eliminate the trans fats.** Donate stick margarine or vegetable shortening (e.g., Crisco) you already have to a food bank or shelter. Instead, use butter for baking. Check your cookies, breads, crackers, chips, and other snacks to make sure they don't contain trans fats. Many national brands now make trans fat–free snack foods, so swap out gradually; no matter what your budget, you can make improvements. Aim for progress, not perfection!

Congratulations, you're doing great! And you've done so much of the heavy lifting already—and lightened yourself in the process. You're well on your way to reaping big savings with your new lifestyle. Now that we've tackled all the elements that go into the state of your plate, let's revisit our snack habits once and for all.

CHAPTER 12

CHOOSING CLEANER FUELS: SNACKS AND "FOOD PRODUCTS"

"Only the power of enlightened business can save the world . . . until commerce is harnessed for the benefit of the planet, the planet doesn't stand a chance.**"**

—Gary Hirshberg, president and CEO, Stonyfield Farm

YOUR LEAN AND GREEN PRESCRIPTION
Enjoy two sustainable snacks a day (100 to 175 calories each)

INCLUDE
Any foods on any Lean and Green Prescription list

Any food from "Your Guide to Sustainable Snacking" on page 40
Limit or avoid: Any foods or "food products" not on either of these lists

It's been hard not to notice that the modern idea of "supermarket" has undergone a radical transformation in the past 20 years. What was once a place to purchase staple ingredients for from-scratch cooking increasingly resembles a cross between a convenience store and a NASA food lab—filled with partially prepared items that require minimal prep time, highly processed products in seemingly outer-space-ready shrink-wrap, pre-portioned foods in individual serving sizes, and "grab-and-go" meals neatly stockpiled in disposable containers. These "foods" have become the new normal.

With 30,000 to 40,000 products lining the shelves in an average supermarket, and roughly 20,000 new products each year vying to break into that space, the choices can be staggering.

To make them appear healthier and gain a market advantage (and often charge more), many new products are now fortified with different combinations of vitamins, minerals, antioxidants, and exotic ingredients. Even products your grandmother probably would have deemed "junk food" are being spun as an indulgence you've earned, a break from your day, or some other euphemism designed to assuage your guilt and convince you that this food fits into your life.

Somewhere.

The American ideal has always defined "progress" as more choices, more options. More is better. But when it comes to food, might there be a tipping point? Have we reached it?

I believe this "food clutter" has sprawled to the point where it's overwhelming us in every way. So many choices are paralyzing rather than empowering. They're clogging our kitchen cabinets, our minivans, our arteries, and now we see they're clogging the atmosphere with carbon. Our kids, seeing stacks of snack foods and cookies in the pantry, revolt against "dinner" and beg and plead for something else, knowing that if they just hold out long enough, an exhausted parent will "give in," throw up the flag, and finally open up those pretzels, that cereal, or whatever else will end the drama.

From what I see around me with family and friends, and from what I hear from clients behind my closed office door, more and more of us are feeling overwhelmed and exhausted by all of this choice and abundance. It's hurting our quality of life, and it's deeply hurting our relationship to food. This isn't eating, it's madness.

Oceans of packaging that required vast amounts of gasoline and other fossil fuels to make it as "easy" for the consumer as possible. Piles of plastic wrappers, microwave bowls, single servings of chocolate cake, breakfast bars to go, and zappable "cheese"—all designed to make a 3-minute eating experience possible. Suddenly, realigning a diet to be healthy and greener seems like it should be astoundingly simple, easy, and straightforward.

So while industrial food has invaded practically every food group and meal of the day, let's make it simple again. The goal of this book, in fact, is to put easy, clean, and delicious food back onto your plate. So let's consider snacks again for a moment.

Believe it or not, snacks are key to just about any successful weight loss plan. As I've said, the right snack can stave off hunger, keep your energy stable throughout the day, and help shave pounds from your waistline by keeping you out of the "hunger danger zone."

But, like most things, there is a dark side to snacks as well. Load up on too much of the wrong kind of snack, and you'll find yourself packing on the pounds, zapped of energy, and wondering why you feel like crap. You see, it all depends on what you're noshing.

I usually recommend that my clients eat two snacks a day, but do what works best for you (occasionally I have clients who aren't snackers; they do just fine by focusing only on the three meals). Personally, I need to snack, as do many of my clients. If that sounds like you too, then read on.

There are two easy tips for leveraging snacking to your advantage: Stick to real food, and keep it to roughly what fits in the palm of your hand.

See what it comes back to? The right foods in the right amounts. Snacking can be a valuable strategy to getting lean if you use it this way. Thinking of snacks as a place where junk food "fits" into your diet is a quick way to end up with a case of carbon and belly bloat.

First, review the section titled "Cool Hot Spot #2: Start Snacking Sustainably" on page 34. That will give you the basics, as well as a complete sustainable snacking list. In addition, here are a few pointers.

- **Don't forgo fat and fiber.** Snacks that pack a bit of fat and fiber will fight hunger best. Research suggests that adding fat or fiber to your snack helps trigger the release of cholecystokinin, a hormone associated with satiety.[1]

- **Remember that protein provides staying power.** Be sure to include some protein in your snack to help delay hunger longer. French researchers found that a high-protein snack kept study participants fuller nearly 40 minutes longer than those whose snack was high carb, while the high-carb snackers got hungry as quickly as the subjects who had no snack at all.[2]

- **Make it last.** Pack a snack that takes a bit longer to eat, so your brain has some time to catch up. I love pistachios in the shell for this! Or things like spreading hummus on a pita, or mashing a hard-cooked egg with salt and pepper, or dip with crackers. Or spreading peanut butter on apple wedges. If you crave ritual, be sure to create one.

- **Go big.** If you are a person who really likes to eat volume, then choose foods that deliver large volume with fewer calories, such as a cup of cubed watermelon, cantaloupe, a fresh salad loaded with super-low-calorie veggies like mushrooms, or air-popped popcorn. They take a lot longer to eat for the same amount of calories than, say, a chocolate doughnut hole or a few french fries.

- **Reach for "health packs" instead of "snack packs."** Make "health packs" by preportioning into reusable containers your own snacks of healthy foods from the sustainable snacking list. Stick to the ones at room temp on the days you have no access to a fridge (e.g., nuts, seeds, dried fruits), and bring the ones that need chillin' on the days you have access to a fridge (e.g., hard-cooked eggs, yogurt or cottage cheese, hummus). This is a much healthier strategy for you and the planet.

Question for you: Have you ever watched any other animal in nature try to procure its food? If not, it might be a worthwhile exercise to bring into sharp focus just how out of whack our current food environment is with our natural biology. I recently went fishing in Wyoming with my dad; we watched as a hawk expended a tremendous amount of energy hovering, flapping, diving and missing, then diving again. This went on for a good 20 minutes. Even my 3-year-old commented on how much work it was. Then finally, pow, a fish in its talons. Up in the tree, then back to the river again to repeat the whole process.

Now contrast that with modern living at its best—sliding into your car, going to the drive-thru, and resting comfortably in your car while someone on the other end hands you an 1,100-calorie meal or a 500-calorie "snack." Hmm.

TOP SIX REASONS PEOPLE SABOTAGE A SNACK

■ They get too hungry before having a snack.

■ They don't pack a healthy option and become victim to the vending machine.

■ They choose a low-fiber or low-fat snack, and hunger returns sooner.

■ They have strong visual cues (e.g., staring at their coworker's candy jar all day is pure torture).

■ They eat directly out of a carton, container, or package. (It's a surefire way to convince yourself you've eaten less than you really have.)

■ They're eating for reasons other than hunger (boredom, procrastination, depression).

If any of these sound like you, take steps to modify your behavior or environment. If you're eating for reasons other than hunger, it is critical that you address the underlying issue or find an outlet other than food if you are to be successful. That's an entire other book in itself.

One thing is clear: Our natural biology makes it extremely difficult to handle a high-calorie eating option with the flick of the wrist or the zap of a microwave button day after day. Of course we're going to gain weight if we have easy access to calorie-dense foods all the time. This, in essence, is the fundamental challenge of all this fast food and "food product" that lines our shelves and our lives these days.

And "diet foods," in my opinion, don't seem all that much better, creating as much carbon and confusion as the regular products (although companies will rarely ever actually use the "d" word). I have counseled many well-intentioned clients who were practically living on portion-controlled frozen dinners, diet sodas, calorie-controlled snack packs, and sugar-free desserts. They certainly were trying to do the right thing, but the only thing I really saw being lightened with all of these "solutions" was people's wallets. Again, ask yourself: If all of these foods *worked,* Americans would be thinner, right?

Most of what is sitting in the center aisles of the supermarket these days is what I call industrial food. While there are certainly exceptions, here are the reasons why it's problematic for these foods to comprise much of your diet.

- Industrial food tends to have a higher calorie density and a lower nutrient density. (Think of the journey of a fresh peach versus a canned peach—less fiber, less vitamin C, and more sugar added in the syrup—moving into a peach pie—more sugar, more saturated or trans fat, and higher calories.)

- Industrial food lacks the vibrant health benefits of fresh, live food. We know the power of real food to provide powerful antioxidants and anti-inflammatory benefits, but so far science hasn't lived up to its promise of simply fortifying foods with these nutrients and getting the exact same benefits.

- Industrial food tends to contain cheaper ingredients that don't contribute to and may even undermine good health

WHAT IS "INDUSTRIAL FOOD"?

Nearly all food passes through some sort of processing before it comes to you, even the most elemental foods such as eggs, lettuce, or nuts. Then there are foods that are lightly processed, say frozen broccoli spears, raisins, a bag of dried beans, a can of stewed tomatoes, or a jar of all-natural peanut butter.

While the exact line of crossover between light and heavier processing is certainly subjective, when I say "industrial food," I am referring to foods that:

■ Have been processed and manipulated in a significant way by the food industry to be easily ready to eat by the consumer

■ Are heavily fortified as opposed to rich in naturally occurring nutrients

■ Are highly preserved or packaged so they don't grow mold until the next millennium (okay, I'm exaggerating a bit, but you get the point)

■ Contain a list of ingredients that are difficult to pronounce, that read like a chemist's shopping list, or that may be of questionable nutritional value (e.g., partially hydrogenated oils, high fructose corn syrup, artificial sweeteners, food coloring and dyes, etc.)

■ Are engineered to deceive our senses with powerful sweet, salty, or flavored tastes that are like crack to our primitive brains

■ Are heavily cross-marketed with things such as Web site games, blogs, MySpace pages, movie tie-ins, and the like

(for example, trans fats or highly refined sweeteners such as high-fructose corn syrup).

■ Industrial food fights our natural biology: It is easy to access, often ready to eat in a second, and available in the car or at the movies—places where you shouldn't be eating. It makes high calorie density too easy, and it makes it too easy to eat a large amount of calories in a small amount of time.

I'm about to say something extremely unpopular in the food business. Take less. Starting now. You can do it. As the authors of the best-selling *Skinny Bitch* quipped, "You cannot keep shoveling the same crap into your mouth and expect to lose weight." To which I would add: "And you can't keep taking as much from the system and wasting as much and successfully trim your carbon footprint."

Cutting back on the wrong kind of snacks, cutting back on overly convenient high-calorie food products, and adding the right amounts of fresh, whole foods are part of the answer for both.

GREEN BENEFITS

The amount of industrialized food that you choose to eat is one of the biggest determinants of your dietary lifestyle. Here's why realigning the amount of processed foods you eat can reap such significant, immediate carbon savings. As I've mentioned before, our food production system consumes about 19 percent of the total amount of energy used in the United States. Nearly a third of that amount is used for *processing and packaging*.[3] Then there is waste; after all, you basically tear open these foods and then throw away the packaging immediately. Ironically, according to the EPA, about one-third of all your trash is packaging, too.

Even more interesting, a landmark 2002 study estimated that up to a third of the total energy in your food footprint is related to snacks, sweets, and drinks, items with little nutritional value.[4] In fact, when I asked Gidon Eshel, one of the researchers, to first quantify the carbon impact of eating meat in relation to the impact of the cars we drive, he emphasized that "trimming industrial food" was the second most powerful way to cut your carbon food footprint after eating fewer animal foods. A growing call from health professionals and "food ecologists" seems to agree.

"Foods that lie to our senses are one of the most challenging features of the Western diet," noted Michael Pollan in his book *In Defense of Food*. Hmmm. Just as all roads lead to Rome, all low-carbon roads seem to lead away from a reliance on processed foods.

I am definitely not suggesting that we simply remove industrial food from American life as a cure-all to our health or environmental ills. Certainly, some industrial food plays a valuable role in our society. In their best forms, they offer convenience to time-strapped Americans, provide valuable shortcuts in the kitchen that help mom or dad get a healthy dinner on the table quickly, and are an essential buffer against possible natural disasters or agricultural failures (think Hurricane Katrina, flooding in Iowa, or a Florida frost that wipes out an entire crop of citrus). And big industry has the clout to make sweeping changes in how Americans eat for the better. For instance, they have helped bring different lettuces (such as mesclun mix, mâche, and arugula) into the mainstream. Big box retailers have also helped create a larger market for organic food, bringing it to a price point that's more within reach of all Americans as opposed to just hippies and yuppies.

But industrial food is slowly taking over our supermarkets and our diets, and has crept into every corner of our lives, from the cereal bars we gobble each morning as we run out the door to the chips we nibble in front of the TV at night. We are eating less food and more "food products." The pendulum has shifted to where the benefit and value that industrial food has to offer is now eclipsed by its sheer volume in our lives, its unhealthy impact on our weight and health, and (as we are now realizing) the significant contributions that this type of food is making in a very real way to global warming.

Industrial food usually has a higher carbon footprint because:

- Consolidation of the food industry has led to fewer players producing more food with a longer life cycle. As a result, food often racks up a big carbon résumé between ingredients, processing, packaging, central distribution, storage, and delivery to point of purchase.

- Industrial food needs to be highly packaged to survive storage and transportation, and to get into the hands of consumers with minimal risk of food-borne illness or contamination.

- Some categories of industrial food (e.g., frozen dinners) require large amounts of fossil fuels to prepare, are then held frozen until you buy them, and then require energy to cook them again—creating a "double warming" effect.

■ If you consider the extensive research and development, marketing, and advertising facet of industrial food (which is by far the lion's share of all food marketing dollars), the carbon footprint becomes even larger.

Of course, even if you shop regularly at a natural foods store, you're bound to notice hundreds of new food products there, too. Many come from "big organic" companies, but looking at the issues of industrial food, it's logical to wonder if food from those "big organic" companies is any better for the planet. Interestingly enough, if you dig around the Internet, you'll quickly discover that most brands in the "organic/natural/healthy" category are actually children of a much larger parent company. If you consider that General Mills owns the Cascadian Farms and Muir Glen Organics lines; Hain Celestial is the company behind Earth's Best Organic Baby Food, Arrowhead Mills, and Walnut Acres; and Kellogg owns Kashi and Morningstar Farms, you begin to realize how intertwined big business is with the organic/healthy market.

So is it any greener to buy from "big organic" companies than to support something smaller and local? Aren't the business realities of bringing large amounts of food consistently to a national market going to require a heavy carbon load, despite lofty-sounding brand names? Is it greenwashing? Indeed, this is one of the thorniest issues in the debate around the proliferation of large-scale organic or natural food companies.

In my opinion, big organic or "clean packaged" foods are still both a great choice for your pantry, and here's why. As Stonyfield Farm president and CEO Gary Hirshberg said, "Business is the only force powerful enough to save the world for my grandchildren."[8] He's right, for even very small improvements in the carbon footprint of large global companies (who make up sizeable portions of total grocery sales) are going to have a much vaster impact on global emissions than the "carbon neutral" efforts of small, mom-and-pop organic labels.

IS BULK A BETTER BUY?

Not necessarily. Buying from a big box retailer is still a gray area when it comes to being green, and it may make it more difficult to get lean. Here's a breakdown.

ISSUE	IS BULK/BIG BOX BETTER?	WHY
Cost	Yes, *if* . . . (see next column)	• Bulk can save you up to 50 percent or more, but only *if* you're not eating the product faster as a result. (I've read dozens of blogs from moms who've noticed that when they load up on a snack because it's on sale, their family plows through the larger amount at the same rate they did the smaller.) If this sounds familiar, proceed with caution. • Big box retailers can also make organics more affordable.
Lean benefit	No	• Larger containers or portions encourage you to eat more.[5] • Your natural satiety cues are readily overridden by food cues such as large portions, easy access, and a highly appealing food.[6] • Even if food tastes junky, you'll eat more if it's in a big container.[7] • Research suggests "buy one get one free" promotions may also encourage you to eat more (blog postings seem to agree).
Green benefit	Bulk bins: Yes	• Buying grains, dried fruit and beans, nuts, and other dry goods from bulk bins in your supermarket or co-op is a greener bite (and leaner, too).
Green benefit	Big box retailers: Probably not	• While you may be cutting down on packaging waste, many of the big bulk suppliers have longer distribution chains. • You're logging an extra shopping trip to go there. • When there's more food, you're likely to waste more. • Bulk fresh items such as hummus, salsa, or produce may spoil before you can use it all.
To Make Sure Buying in Bulk Doesn't Just Mean You Eat More		• Pre-portion single servings from large containers. • Avoid stockpiling trigger foods or high-risk foods. • Replenish on a set schedule, so if it gets eaten faster, that's it for now. • Use your bulk bins in your supermarket or co-op. • Think before you buy.

THE GROWING PROBLEM OF "GREENWASHING"

What's the definition of "green"? Right now, it's a virtual free-for-all. "Green labeling" regulations are still loose and undefined, with the Federal Trade Commission (FTC) still just taking comments on the issue. This makes it harder for you to know who's "greenwashing" their products and who is genuinely doing better by the Earth.

In the meantime, some companies are acting independently to define, measure, and report sustainability. However, while many of these companies may measure the same "what," they vary in how they measure "how," which makes direct comparisons difficult. So read the fine print carefully.

To be fair, some companies are also wary to invest when "green technology" is changing so fast. They are still not sure how much the consumer is willing to pay for "greener" food, and the return to the company seems a distinct shade of gray.

So here's my advice on how to minimize your exposure to "greenwashing":

■ Use Your L.E.A.N. Cheat Sheet (see page 154) to decide whether the product meets your basic green criteria.

If American consumers leverage the power of the purse, history shows that food companies will respond (Exhibit A: low fat or low carb). When you switch to cleaner packaged foods (which is where all of these healthier companies fall), your purchases send a powerful message to companies about what sort of business models you will support, and what kind of "food world" you want to live in.

It's not a perfect solution, but it's a better solution. But as I said, it's not a cure-all. Just as with every other aspect of the global warming crisis, we can't simply shop our way out of it by switching to greener choices. While it is tempting to think that you can nourish your body and your social conscience at the same time as a consumer, remember that commercial food, even organic, is still one of the most resource-heavy areas of your diet (those organic chicken nuggets or potato chips, for instance). Part of the underlying problem

■ Look for a clean ingredient list and eco-chic labels (such as Fair Trade, Sustainably Harvested, Bird Friendly, and Organic).

■ Look for minimal packaging (not excessive) that's made from a high percentage of recycled materials, if possible.

■ Keep in mind that glass, metal, and ceramic containers, from a sheer environmental impact, are greener choices than plastic. If you do have to choose plastic, check the number: plastics #1, #2, #4, and #5 are safest for you and the planet (and #1 and #2 are the most commonly recycled). Things that are reusable (e.g., reusable glass milk bottles) are some of the greenest overall choices if you can find them. This is another benefit to looking local.

■ Remember that the heavier the item, the more fuel it requires to transport.

■ Lastly, use your head—and your nose. Does it look or smell like greenwashing to you (bottled water from another continent that claims to be "carbon negative," for example)?

with our plate (and cup) is simply how big it is. Take less. It's critical that you realign your equation here to be more in balance with calorie needs, which for most of us will automatically help realign the amount of resources we use.

TAKE ACTION NOW

For any remaining items in your pantry that we haven't already tackled in another chapter, use this guide to decide whether to keep or toss (meaning, donate to a food pantry or charity).

■ **Keep it short.** Read the label; the fewer ingredients, the better. This is because each ingredient has its own carbon footprint before it even enters into your food (and is often

KNOW YOUR LOCAL RECYCLING SITUATION

While the "lean" piece is wrapped up once you've eaten your food, the "green" issues linger to the trash can and well beyond. How to be sure you continue to reduce your carbon footprint? "The best thing consumers can do is to know their local recycling and composting infrastructure," advised Chad Smith, a sustainability and packaging expert for Earthbound Farms Organics, when I called him to ask for his thoughts. "That will help you make the right decisions, because you'll know which materials to look for when you're purchasing."

Packaging made with post-consumer (recycled) paper may have some carbon savings, but bioplastics—corn-based plastics that promise to be compostable—seem to be more uncertain. Smith, whose company has looked extensively at whether or not to adopt these bioplastics as "greener answers," says there are currently some drawbacks. "There's a lot of interest right now in corn-based plastics, but a lot of these don't necessarily biodegrade unless they have the exact conditions (which means you better be tending that home compost carefully); and because they are only compostable under certain conditions; at the end of the day they're not necessarily a win for the Earth."

If you live in a city with curbside composting (such as San Francisco, but

---

produced somewhere else). So bread made with "flour, salt, yeast, and water" will likely have a smaller carbon footprint than bread made with a litany of ingredients, each with its own footprint.

- **Keep it simple.** The ingredient list shouldn't read like a chemist's shopping list. If you can't pronounce everything and do not know what the ingredients are, be sure to put that item in the pile of food to donate.

- **Keep it clean.** Avoid products with high-fructose corn syrup, trans fats, and artificial sweeteners. Minimize refined white flour (called "wheat" flour) and opt for whole grains instead. Minimize stabilizers, colorings, preservatives, and other ingredients that wouldn't be found in your home kitchen. Less is more.

not my town of Park City), where "green waste" is collected along with regular recyclables such as plastics and paper, then there's a chance those compostable plastics may actually end up being converted to the soil. However, if you just toss it into your recycling bin (as I did prior to my interview with Chad, thinking I was doing the right thing), these bioplastics can end up polluting the recyclable plastic stream, or else go to the landfill. Oops. So know before you buy.

Right now the burden of the end product has been borne by *you*, the consumer: You have to recycle it; your town has to figure out how to handle all of the waste; and your taxes reflect the decisions of your elected officials. The idea of "extended producer responsibility" is taking hold in Europe and has already created significant changes in the packaging scene. In the future, "producer responsibility" in the United States may well be extending to the taking back, recovery, and final disposal of the product. This policy, if implemented in the United States (it's been in place in much of the UK since the 1990s), would shift the end-of-life costs of collecting, sorting, and managing post-consumer packaging that are typically borne by localities to the producers of packaged goods.

- **Pare down the packaging.** How your food is packaged imparts a "double warming" effect on your food's carbon footprint, first when it is produced, then when it's thrown away (recycling is good, but it still takes energy). One layer of packaging is better than two, so see if you can find a less heavily packaged choice instead. The higher the recycled content of the packaging, the better. Another easy, immediate strategy is to eliminate as many "single-serving" items as you can, including juice boxes, string cheese, snack packs, chips bags, hot chocolate packs, and cereal boxes. It takes 2 seconds to portion these out yourself at home using storage containers, sippy cups, or zip-top bags.
- **Concentrate if you can.** According to a report in the *National Geographic* 2008 Green Guide, concentrated juices

are hands down greener because of all the carbon savings of shipping a smaller, lighter package. Extend that logic to things such as buying bouillon cubes or concentrate instead of broths, and tea bags instead of bottled tea beverages.

- **Go a deeper shade of green.** Subscribe to *National Geographic*'s Green Guide at www.thegreenguide.com. The Green Guide is chock-full of simple, useful ideas, broken down into achievable steps, and regularly covers food and food packaging issues.

- **Consider second use.** While every packaging choice (e.g., glass or plastic) has trade-offs, the final carbon count depends on what you do with it. Reuse is roughly 93 percent more efficient than recycling, so choose food in packages you know you can somehow reuse, or at the very least can recycle. The carbon footprint of an aluminum can versus plastic versus cardboard, for instance, is significantly related to whether or not it gets recycled. And the vast majority don't.

- **Clear away the clutter.** Just as you clean out your closet, you need to purge your pantry. Donate any food items you haven't used in a year. You know what I'm talking about— the random cans of soup a relative left behind on her last visit, that cake flour you tried baking with once but never used again. Toss anything that's expired. Be ruthless, really ruthless.

- **Cut the crap.** Once your pantry is purged, be vigilant about not stockpiling food, especially snack food, junk food, or trigger foods. Stockpiling food doesn't seem to create savings. More options encourage you to eat more and waste more, and ultimately they cost you more. At most, I recommend keeping the following on hand: one type of cookie, two or three types of breakfast cereal, one or two boxes of crackers, and one dessert in the freezer. Rotate through family favorites if meeting different requests is a challenge in your house.

PART V

WHITTLE YOUR WAISTLINE WITH SUSTAINABLE SIPPING

Congratulations! You've tackled practically everything that's on your plate. If you've followed the "Take Action Now" steps and been greening your pantry along the way, you're no doubt already reaping the rewards of leaner living. Great job.

Now that you've completed your eco-makeover on your pantry and fridge, we'll also move from your plate to your glass to get you on the road to sipping more sustainably.

So sit back, relax, pour a glass of your favorite red wine (in Chapter 13 you'll find out whether you should make it from California or France), a local microbrew—or a nonalcoholic drink if you do not consume alcohol—and savor for a moment what you have accomplished. As this next section gets you drinking responsibly for your health and the planet, you might as well be drinking deliciously while you read.

GET STARTED NOW: REAL SIMPLE SOLUTIONS TO START LOSING TODAY

1 **DRINK RESPONSIBLY: THE TWO W'S THAT SHOULD BE IN YOUR GLASS.** Ditch all your bottled beverages, even the diet ones. Purified tap water, brewed coffee, and tea are your mainstay brews from now on for a cleaner, leaner, greener you from the inside out with zero calories and much fewer fossil fuel calories than their bottled brethren. If you can afford the extra calories, wine in moderation helps keep you super healthy and enriches your life in other ways, too.

2 **SUSTAINABLE SPLURGES: CHOCOLATE IS A SPLURGE THAT'S WORTH IT TO YOUR HEALTH AND TO THE PLANET.** The key is to nibble this and other "green treats" the right way.

CHAPTER 13

WATER, WINE, AND JUICE

Sip Your Way to Slim with the Greenest Glass

"A chilled plastic bottle of water in the convenience store cooler is the perfect symbol of this moment in American commerce and culture. It acknowledges our demand for instant gratification . . . and our token concern for health. Its packaging and its transport depend entirely on cheap fossil fuel."

—Charles Fishman, journalist, *Fast Company*, 2007

YOUR LEAN AND GREEN PRESCRIPTION
zero-calorie beverages (Eat your calories, don't drink them.)

ENJOY DAILY

Unlimited filtered or purified tap water

Fresh brewed coffee or tea (especially green, black, or herbal)

IF YOU CAN AFFORD THE CALORIES

Up to 6 ounces 100 percent fruit or vegetable juice

Up to one (5-ounce) glass of wine a day for women, up to two glasses for men

LIMIT

Sports drinks (unless you are an athlete exercising more than 60 minutes a day and not looking to lose weight)

Designer coffee drinks on the go

Yogurt drinks and commercially made smoothies (unless you can afford the extra calories and the ingredient list is clean)

AVOID

Bottled water

Canned or bottled sodas (even diet), juice blends, diet drinks, health waters, and all of the hundreds of "hybrid" drinks on the market

Any juice drink that isn't 100 percent juice

Any drinks with artificial sweeteners

Energy drinks

Milkshakes

Single-serving or highly packaged beverages

Beer and spirits

For many people, the biggest obstacle to weight loss may be sitting in their *glass* rather than on their plate. Are you nursing a cup of something or other all day? Texting your barista? Deciding that 4:00 is the "new" 5:00 when it comes to pouring an acceptable glass of wine?

If so, then listen up. According to the 2004 scientific report that was the basis of the 2005 US Dietary Guidelines, "Available prospective studies suggest a positive association between the consumption of sugar-sweetened beverages and weight gain. A reduced intake of added sugars (especially sugar-sweetened beverages) may be helpful in achieving recommended intakes of nutrients and in weight control."[1]

If that's too techie for you, consider how one of my sassier clients put it: "The size of your glass determines the size of your ass."

Here's the skinny on getting lean: Liquid calories have to go. Or at least go down. A lot. How easy, because it's one of the clearest and most precise overlaps with a greener diet as well.

The research is clear. Liquid calories do *not* register in your brain the same way that food calories do, which means your body doesn't recognize them and adjust your intake accordingly. People who drink a lot of liquid calories tend to weigh more than people who don't.[2] Think you're okay with diet drinks? Think again. Drinking diet soda has not been shown to help you lose weight; it may even contribute to weight gain.[3]

Perhaps more alarming is that our children are learning that tap water is something to be shunned, that designer coffee concoctions resembling caffeinated milkshakes are an acceptable (if expensive) late afternoon "pick-me-up," and that there is no health downside to slurping on a sea of liquid calories all day long. And as you'll soon see, the packaging coming from all these beverages is staggering. It's the perfect storm for your hips, and it's adding tons of carbon to your personal plume.

Water

If things such as fish are murky, thank goodness beverages are crystal clear. Drink cleanly. Skip the beverage aisle, and you'll start trimming immediately. Stick to nature's best—purified water.

I'm sure the lean benefits of water are rather obvious, but here's a quick review: Drinking water helps keep your skin looking great, your GI tract healthy and regular, your energy levels and focus maximized, your munchies at bay, your workouts going strong, and toxins flushed from your system, plus a host of other benefits. It's made by nature, and it's a renewable resource. Plus, it's zero calories, so there's no weight gain, which is especially important because liquid calories don't register with your brain. As for other beverages, if you can afford the extra calories, small amounts of 100 percent fruit or vegetables juice and wine can provide numerous health benefits, too. I'll give you a lot more direction on the best coffee and tea choices in the next chapter, but feel free to enjoy those, either hot or cold, as well.

So how much water do you really need? The answer may surprise you. While drinking water regularly throughout the day is a sound strategy, if you drink water, coffee, or tea with meals and snacks, plus anytime you feel thirst coming on, chances are you're well hydrated.

Contrary to popular belief, you don't need to force down 8 to 10 glasses of water *in addition* to all your other food and drink choices. In fact, researchers have recently taken a closer look at the myths around water intake and found that very little was based in actual science. The latest guidelines from the Institute of Medicine (IOM) state that "the vast majority of healthy people adequately meet their daily hydration needs by letting thirst be their guide."[4]

Another easy way to see if you need to drink more water is to do a quick urine check—it should be clear and have no odor (as opposed to being darker with a strong smell). A few exceptions to this rule: Children, the elderly, and people who are ill should not let thirst be their guide because they may not have fully functioning thirst responses. Likewise, those at high altitudes, in very hot temperatures, or exercising hard for a long time may need more water than thirst dictates.

If you're a regular soda or beer drinker, switching to water can be one of the easiest ways to lose weight fast. Several years ago, I was counseling firefighters and police officers throughout the state of Massachusetts. In the first days of our meetings, I brought in my "sugar tubes" showing how much sugar (about 10 teaspoons) is in a 12-ounce can of soda. Several of these guys were drinking two or three cans of soda a day! That visual alone was enough to get a couple of the guys to stop cold turkey, and the results were fast and furious. A few lost about 20 pounds in 6 months! I've seen similar results for nightly beer drinkers, too. Check out the table below for some other examples of the poundage you can lose by cutting back on your brews.

DRINKING RESPONSIBLY GETS YOU ON THE FAST TRACK TO LEAN

CUT OUT THIS	FOR THIS MANY CALORIES	AND LOSE THIS MANY POUNDS IN A YEAR
12-oz beer a night	150	15
3 (5 oz each) glasses of wine a week	300	4.5
12-oz soda each day	150	15
2 Starbucks venti lattes (using 2% milk) a week	480	7
12-oz Gatorade (Performance Series) after workouts 4 nights a week	1,240	18.5

GREEN BENEFITS

After beef, bottled water may represent the single biggest, fastest change you can make to shrink your carbon footprint. In the cluttered beverage aisle these days it's easy to forget that all this stuff is completely unnecessary.

Next time you're in the supermarket, take a good hard look at the beverage and juice aisle. You'll see the immense "cost of convenience" in action, to your waistline *and* your waste-line. That daily love affair with your barista, office vending machine, or smoothie bar can add up, too: Cups, lids, straws, napkins, stirrers, coffee sleeves, and all the other accessories you get nowadays affect not only price but also the carbon footprint of your brew.

You see, premade beverages do several things: They foster an increased desire for sweetness, add big bucks to your food bill, pack lots of extra weight onto your shopping trips (which means more gasoline needed to pull them home), and come in overwhelming levels of packaging.

Of course, the nutritionist in me absolutely sees the benefits of zero-calorie beverages. Flavored waters, diet sodas, seltzers, and other low-calorie or zero-calorie sweetened beverages can add flavor and variety to a diet without pouring on extra calories. They keep life flexible and fun. And they free up some more calories to go back on your *plate*. So zero-calorie is certainly a better choice if your sole goal is lean. But this book is about the intersection of personal and planetary health, and here's another green truth: Zero-calorie doesn't mean zero-impact.

First drawback: Liquid is one of the heavier types of food calories to ship, so it requires more fuel to transport than many, many other areas of your diet. That's why "drinking responsibly" begins to take on a whole new meaning.

Second drawback: the packaging. If every human being on the planet adopted the average American's drinking habits, we'd need another planet to sustain it, and quickly. Every *second* Americans toss 694 plastic bottles, totaling more than 60 million a day, and every day we dispose of 100 million aluminum steel cans (that's enough to build a roof over all of New York City).[5] Since less than 30 percent of those products are recycled, it creates a glut in our waste streams and has a "double warming" effect of breaking down into planet-warming gases.

Luckily, the solution is easy. Simply put, bottled water is choking the planet with both greenhouse gases and trash. When you drink it, you land squarely in the hot zone. While it's pretty much "ditto" for the rest of the beverage aisle (excluding the exceptions I made above), we'll concentrate on the issues as they pertain to water. Just keep in mind that they ring true for other packaged beverages as well.

In 2006, Americans guzzled more than 31 *billion* liters of bottled water, shelling out more than $15 billion in the process—more than they spent on iPods or movie tickets.[6] That's perfectly good money that you can now put toward your new green cuisine. And that's 28 gallons of water for every man, woman, and child living in America, water that required more than 900,000 *tons* of plastic to manufacture all those bottles to bring it to you. And who knows how many of those were chillin' in a nice 40°F cooler in a mini mart, the airport, or the food court before you decided to buy them?

In the United States alone, roughly 1 billion bottles of water are shipped around the country each week in ships, trains, and trucks; that's equivalent to a weekly convoy of 37,800 18-wheelers delivering something we could get for *much* less fossil fuel simply by turning on the tap. What's more, it's a fast-growing category. Flavored water sales alone have climbed 35 percent since 2005.

Gulp. Want some more? Here are some other facts that I personally find hard to swallow.

- According to the Earth Policy Institute, the annual fossil fuel footprint of bottled water consumption in the United States is equivalent to more than 50 million barrels of oil—enough to run 3 million cars for 1 year.[7]

- Just manufacturing the roughly 30 billion plastic bottles used for water in the United States each year requires the equivalent of more than 17 million barrels of crude oil; transporting these bottles and selling them from chilled machines can double that, depending on where you live.

- Almost 40 percent of all US bottled water sales is just filtered tap water—*water that is already perfectly safe to drink*—sold at a premium. It's bottled in petroleum-rich plastic and shipped around the country.

- The United States is the world's number-one guzzler of bottled water, despite having the absolute safest water supply in the world (one out of six people in the world has no dependable, safe drinking water).

- Americans are actually paying up to four times as much per gallon for their designer H_2O as they are for gasoline, and about 1,000 times more than they pay for tap water.

- "Lighter bottles, carbon offsets, carbon negative"—these are all shades of greenwashing when it comes to water. At the end of the day, we can get water in a much greener, cheaper, and equally safe way—the tap.

PAYING MORE FOR BOTTLED WATER THAN OIL[8]

ITEM	COST PER LITER*	COST PER GALLON*
Fiji	$2.08	$7.90
Dasani	$1.29	$4.90
Aquafina	$1.59	$6.04
Regular unleaded gasoline		$4.08
Average municipal water supply		$0.01

*Water prices from Shaw's Supermarket, 71 Dodge Street, Beverly, MA 01915, on June 17, 2008.

Ironically, 30 years ago, bottled water barely existed as a market. Today, Americans drink more bottled water than anyone in the world—at an immense cost to the planet and our own pocketbooks.

If you don't like the taste of your tap water, or want extra insurance that your water is safe, then by all means get a filter. There are some great filters available that can give you fresh-tasting, clean water from your tap, such as a Brita pitcher filter, a PUR filter, or a Culligan Reverse Osmosis (RO) filter that goes right on your faucet.

Is there a carbon cost to tap water, too? Of course. But unless Americans are willing to go without water piped into their homes, their gyms, their offices, and their malls (remember, no piped water means no flush toilets—how likely is *that*?), piped water is a fixed cost that will be there regardless.

Luckily, it seems that people are getting the message. "Back to the Tap" initiatives are filtering across some of the largest cities in the country—with places such as New York City and San Francisco now banning bottled water at meetings of public officials, recognizing that it's quickly filling up precious landfill space and draining tax coffers in one fell swoop.

FIVE WAYS TO MAKE TAP WATER TASTY

■ Fill an ice cube tray with water and then add whole berries. They add gorgeous color, flavor, and antioxidants to your glass. If you can afford the calories, add a splash of 100 percent juice to the cubes as well.

■ In winter, steep some of your favorite herbal tea, cool in the fridge, and add a bit of raw local honey and some citrus wedges for a sustainable and seasonal sipfest.

■ Stir in fresh grated ginger, a mint sprig, and a squeeze of fresh tangerine juice for zing, vitamin C, and digestive health.

■ Think spa water: Float sliced cucumbers or lime for a cleansing, refreshing change.

■ Make a DIY seltzer. If you can't give up the fizz, consider buying a home seltzer machine that lets you turn up the fizz on your tap water. It's much greener than buying, schlepping, and then disposing of all those bottles (and ultimately cheaper, too).

I find that food changes can sometimes be difficult to make for even the most dedicated do-gooder; beverage changes, by comparison, can sometimes be more easily and quickly adapted. Luckily, drinking from the tap in a reusable cup is one of the easiest, quickest ways to cut your carbon footprint and food bill, and drinking water in lieu of high-calorie beverages such as designer coffee drinks, juices, and sodas will have you treading more lightly in other important ways, too—namely your weight.

Bottled water is a wonderful safety net and a lifesaving resource in times of crisis or emergency. In other regions of the world, it is a critical insurance against questionable water sources. But here in the United States, our daily reliance seems symbolic of how careless and wasteful our lifestyles have truly become. Let's make it a habit to leave it where it belongs. Alone.

- Purchase nontoxic, reusable water bottles for you and your family. Stainless steel is another good alternative. Get your kids on board, too, with their own nontoxic eco-friendly water bottles. If you're comfortable using something from your current stash of plastic workout or camping bottles, then by all means do so. You can use one in your car, stash it in your gym bag, or keep one handy at work.

- Bring a glass, mug, or cup to work and ditch the plastic and paper cups by the water cooler.

- Make a tasty antioxidant-rich brew. Brew up a batch of green or herbal tea for a boost of antioxidants and flavor; stick it in the fridge to cool. Garnish with citrus wedges in the winter and berries and mint in the summer.

- Use your existing bottled water *wisely*; save it for critical times rather than consuming it daily.

Now that we've tackled water, let's move on to the other "W" that might be in your glass, wine.

Wine

In 2008, Americans became the number-one wine consumers in the world, surpassing even our wine-loving *amis* in France and Italy. If you enjoy wine, it can remain a healthy and delicious part of your lean and green lifestyle because it has so many positive health benefits and adds a wonderful dimension to the flavor of your meals.

A bottle of wine is alive, teeming with compounds for your health and your heart, not to mention your taste buds. You have probably heard by now that drinking red wine in moderation is a healthy habit; this is because it contains powerful compounds called polyphenols that help keep your heart, brain, and arteries working effectively into ripe old age. A study from the University of Bordeaux found wine drinkers had a 35 percent reduction in death rates from cardiovascular disease, and a 24 percent reduction in death rates from cancer, compared to people who didn't drink wine.[9] Regular, moderate wine drinking also seems to cut your risk of stroke, dementia, and Alzheimer's disease.[10] Think of it as Roto-Rooter for your arteries.

The key here is *moderation:* up to one glass per day for women and up to two for men. Calories climb quickly. A 5-ounce glass of red wine has about 100 calories—about as much as a slice of bread. Even if you are "moderate" all week, but drink several additional glasses over the weekend, you may be imbibing in the caloric equivalent of half a loaf of bread.

So nix the temptation to tell yourself it's "nutritionist-approved" while pouring that second (or third) glass, as there's no additional health benefit. If you're working hard to lose weight but still want to keep the wine in your diet, as many of my clients do, here's the straight talk: To fit in those extra calories, you gotta be exercising. *Really* exercising.

Whatever you do, do not simply cut other foods out, especially healthy foods, in order to make room for wine. You are less likely to shed pounds, and you may be compromising your nutrition, your body's metabolic rate, and your health. Especially if you are postmenopausal, you may find it difficult to maintain your current weight (and even harder to lose weight) if you include alcohol. Be sure to make the rest of your calories count, with nutrient-dense, moderate-calorie choices. If you do choose to include wine, watch your portions and be sure to keep active and exercise.

Note: If you choose not to drink alcohol, you can still reap some of the same cardiovascular benefits by enjoying 4 ounces of 100 percent grape juice every day, which is a great strategy for your kids, too.

Also, just an aside here for readers scouring the chapter looking for a discussion of other alcoholic drinks: Beer and spirits are not officially on my lean and green list. While both, when consumed in modest amounts, have some positive effects on "good"

HDL cholesterol, the Go Green Get Lean Diet promotes wine instead because wine will give you those same benefits *plus* many others. And beer and spirits, like all alcohol, come in high-calorie packages, so they're some of the fastest ways to pack on the pounds. From a green standpoint, the same production, shipping, transportation, and refrigeration (as well as packaging and marketing) issues all apply.

That being said, if you're not a wine drinker *and* you can afford the extra calories (as both beer and spirits are classic "empty calories" from a nutrition and weight standpoint), then wet your whistle with a local microbrew (it's much easier to find local beer dotting the country than it is wine) and use Your L.E.A.N. Cheat Sheet (see page 154) as a guide to greening your cocktail.

GREEN BENEFITS

Sipping a French Bordeaux or a California Cab may be heaven to your arteries and your palate, but which one is better for the planet? The answer may surprise you.

While obvious for the folks living in California or France, the answer becomes murkier for those of us who are landlocked. A 2007 study that looked at the carbon footprint of wine found that because of the weight of shipping glass bottles of liquid, *transportation to the consumer* was the single biggest carbon factor, even over whether or not the wine was organic. Which means that if you live east of Columbus, Ohio, drinking like a "locavore" means it's greener to fill your glass with that French Bordeaux.[11] *Ooh la la.*

Here are a few other tips to keep in mind.

- Magnums are more energy efficient; half bottles are much less efficient.
- Boxed wines are among the most efficient of all.
- Choose standard bottles rather than thicker ones (which you often find at the high-end premium range), because they are more energy efficient.

- Companies that ship wine in bulk closer to the consumer and *then* bottle are greener (this saves on the cost of transporting all the bottles), so when in doubt, ask.
- Buying wine directly from the vineyard is a high-carbon habit, as wineries often overnight cases to clients around the country via air (to minimize temperature fluctuations and ensure product quality).
- Organic, sustainable, or biodynamic wines make a small difference to overall carbon footprint when compared to transportation.

Of course, there are some practical realities to this new approach to choosing the greenest wines, such as the value of the dollar against European currency, for one. Or the marketing challenge of trying to persuade people to unscrew a box cap rather than pop open a cork. My husband, a self-proclaimed oenophile, visibly cringed at

THE GLASS IS ALWAYS GREENER ON THE OTHER SIDE

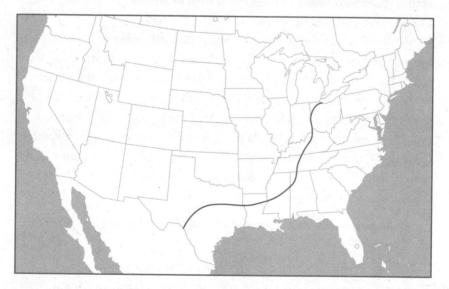

This map shows the approximate break-even point between Bordeaux and Napa wines. If you live west of the line, California wine will likely have a lower carbon footprint. East of the line, and France is a better bet.

CARBON EMISSIONS OF THREE WINES HEADING TO CHICAGO[12]

Boutique Napa winery	4.5 kg/bottle	(overnight air)
France	2.12 kg/bottle	(boat, truck)
Australia	3.44 kg/bottle	(boat, then train or truck)

my suggestion for moving to a wine box in the name of saving the planet. Might people draw a line in the sand at the thought of getting their wine from a milk carton–like container (one of the other suggestions the study authors proposed)? I certainly know a few who would, and I believe I live with one of them. (Heck, if I'm really honest, I may even be one of them.)

You may decide instead that you're more than willing to cut back on a few steaks a year, or to *really* always pass on the bottled water at the office meetings from now on, or to bike to the wine bar instead of drive (probably a better idea anyway) and consider these savings a "balancing out" of your love of wine served the old-fashioned way. After all, the vast health benefits of wine in moderation make it worth including if you can. As for my house, we still drink our wine from a bottle, but we stick to wines from California and Oregon, and are now pairing it with much more vegetarian and green cuisine.

TAKE ACTION NOW

- Check out the US map and see what the greenest option is for you.
- Buy your wine from your local wine shop (ideally, stock up to maximize your personal trip) rather than having it shipped from the Internet or from a mailing list.
- If you live in a wine-producing region, try to sip like a local.
- Buy larger magnums if you can, don't order or buy half bottles, and consider buying wine in a box.

ORGANIC, SUSTAINABLE, AND BIODYNAMIC WINES

Many wineries, from boutique to large well-known brands, are dipping their toes into sustainable, organic, and biodynamic practices, finding that organic agriculture can yield better results for the land and the wine. Most wineries don't necessarily bang the organic drum loudly as a marketing tool, and many don't even mention it on their labels, either because they may not be officially "certified organic," or because they want to compete with the mainstream on the merits of the wine itself rather than be seen in only the "organics" category. While you will still reap health benefits from standard red wine, and these programs may not nudge the carbon count down significantly per se, they certainly provide other numerous benefits to the planet. Here's a quick look at the terms and what they mean.

Sustainable: The wine producer follows a voluntary sustainability program established by the Wine Institute that has a step-by-step guide to "best practices," where producers then receive a sustainability rating of 1 to 4 (4 being the best). So far, more than 1,100 wineries have evaluated their own practices, according to the Wine Institute. One key difference is that the application of synthetic compounds and pesticides is allowed but discouraged.

Organic: Wine has to meet federal organic guidelines and certifications. A very small percentage of vineyards currently have this certification, as it is costly and time-consuming. In addition to farming organically, no sulfur (a key component of the aging process) can be added to the wines.

Biodynamic: An approach to agriculture that treats the soil as a living entity and focuses on balancing the entire system, aligning with nature's cycles, and using natural predator/prey systems. Part mystical, part practical, the philosophy has advocates who claim it brings the soil into perfect alignment, making for delicious and sustainable wine.

Juice

Truly fresh-squeezed fruit or vegetable juice tastes wonderful and can refresh and awaken you. Its live enzymes provide a powerful cocktail of nutrients. And juicing can be a great way to harness the power of foods that have been used medicinally in alternative medicine for centuries (e.g., beet juice for liver cleansing, celery juice for blood pressure, ginger to soothe your stomach).

LEAN BENEFITS

Juice is one of the classic "in moderation can be good for you" foods. For many people, 4 to 6 ounces of 100 percent juice can be a quick, easy, reliable, and nutritious way to sneak in an extra serving of disease-fighting fruits and veggies. And let's face it: Americans are notorious underachievers when it comes to eating enough fruits and veggies; juice offers a valuable shortcut. But as with everything, the right kind, in the right amounts, is key to getting the results you want.

If you can't afford the extra calories, are diabetic, or are especially prone to blood sugar swings, then definitely skip the juice. Eat the whole fruit instead. You'll get more nutrition and phytochemicals in a lower-calorie package, plus loads of fiber, which slims you down and fills you up. The other advantage is that eating the whole fruit will work with your biology and your brain to help you eat less later (remember, liquid calories don't really register with your brain).

Drink cleanly by choosing only 100 percent juice. Once you leave 100 percent juice, it's a slippery slope down to "liquid candy."

For children, stick with no more than 4 to 6 ounces of 100 percent juice per day. More may interfere with appetite, may push out other important beverages such as water and milk, and may be training them to like only sweet drinks. Even the American Academy of Pediatrics issued guidelines in 2001 advising no more than 6 ounces per day for kids, having seen an alarming increase in juice consumption.

Skip the added extras. These include vitamins, immune boosters, and mineral additions. For one thing, the juice is apt to be in a higher-carbon package. Second, you're probably going to pay more for them, and often only small amounts are added for marketing purposes; ignore the hype on the labels and eat a healthy diet instead. Two possible exceptions: calcium (if you don't take a calcium supplement, do not include calcium-rich foods regularly, and are at risk for osteoporosis) and plant stanols (if you have high cholesterol).

Juice still tends to be a high-carbon part of your diet because of the waste associated with it (consider that it typically takes about four oranges to make 6 ounces of juice). And if your juice is made somewhere else and shipped to you (instead of buying it freshly made at a juice bar, for instance), there's the added carbon of shipping heavy liquids. So here's what you need to know for a more sustainable squeeze.

Buy 100 percent frozen juice concentrate as the gold standard, if it's an option. It's the best for nutrition, cost, and significant carbon savings (you're not shipping all that water around).

Stick to American beauties for another winning lean and green overlap (revisit the list of American beauties on page 137 in Chapter 9). Exotic superfruit juices don't give you any more help in soothing American stress, and likely have a higher carbon footprint and a higher price tag. Good old-fashioned Concord grape juice, pomegranate, cherry, and blueberry juice, in contrast, have ample research showing clear health benefits.

Check that OJ label. Avoid buying conventional juice that is grown in tropical areas such as Brazil or Costa Rica. According to the Rainforest Action Network, conventional oranges grown in Brazil and other South American countries are often grown on areas of rainforest that have been burned and cleared to plant these trees, removing a critical "carbon cooler"—a double carbon footprint whammy.

Shop for eco-chic labels. If you do decide to swig more exotic juices, or common juice that's grown in exotic locales, be *extra* sure to sip sustainably and organically, so you're not destroying tropical areas to fuel your zest for some zingy new brew.

Pick minimal packaging. Packaging in this category can be outrageous. Avoid single-serving bottles, juice boxes, and any "power juices" in annoyingly (to me) small sizes in the supermarket, sometimes shrink-wrapped to boot. (I can't help but notice many of these exotic juices come in small bottles—probably so you won't pay attention to how much you're paying per ounce.) This ups the carbon cost of shipping the juice around, because the packaging-to-product ratio is so skewed. So buy in bulk if you can. And juicing yourself will minimize the packaging big time. And, of course, recycle that packaging!

Squeeze it yourself. If you're an OJ or grapefruit junkie, consider investing in a hand-pressed juicer for amazingly fresh flavor, and then start squeezin' the old-fashioned way. It's super easy and kids love it! A great example of quality over quantity, it cuts your carbon footprint and packaging. (Two added pluses: You'll burn a few extra calories while you're at it, and it will be easier to stick to 4 to 6 ounces because you'll be too busy to stand there and squeeze more.)

Soda

How can I put this lightly? Soda sucks.

There is no room for soda, diet soda, "health drinks," or energy drinks on the Go Green Get Lean Diet. Ignore them. There's no nutritional benefit to soda and there are *lots* of nutritional drawbacks: the added empty calories, the fact that they perpetuate a continued drive to seek sweetness, the possible interference with the calcium to phosphorus balance in your body, and their ability to zap your vitality and wreak havoc on your blood sugar. Unlike other high-carbon foods that at least provide a specific and measurable health benefit (e.g., fresh Alaskan salmon, a glass of fresh-squeezed juice), it's harder to salve your eco-guilt by drinking greenwashed diet soda that is manufactured using wind power.

Energy drinks are even worse. Essentially the pimped-out version of sodas, they jack up the calories, the sugar, and the caffeine in a major way. They induce a high-stress state called fight or flight in your body that taxes your adrenal glands and can overwhelm your body's stress response over time. Talk about an immediate place to trim; America's food supply provides about 200 calories per person each day in soft drinks alone, in the form of high-fructose corn syrup. Soft drinks are the single biggest source of added sugars in the American diet today, composing about 33 percent of the carbohydrates in people's diets. No wonder we have a weight problem.

Since 1978, soda consumption in the United States has tripled for boys and doubled for girls. According to the National Soft Drink Association (now renamed a more benign-sounding "American Beverage

Association"), consumption of soft drinks is the equivalent of more than 600 cans (12 ounces each) per American per year. Young males ages 12 to 29 are the biggest consumers at more than 160 gallons per year—that's almost 2 quarts per day.

LEAN BENEFITS

Drink diet soda, get lean, right? Wrong. Most people drink diet soda and "health" beverages to help control their weight. The problem is, the research actually points in the opposite direction—that people drinking these beverages aren't any thinner, and that the more you drink, the more you may actually end up gaining. An 8-year study from the University of Texas found that for diet soda drinkers, the risk of overweight climbed by a whopping 41 percent for subjects who drank one to two diet sodas a day.[13]

To me, this group of products seems a particularly sneaky subset of the soda category. They appeal to your desire to lose weight. They may add a few vitamins, minerals, or exotic ingredients to make them seem healthy and convince you that they provide some advantage over, say, water. They may tempt you with "light" versions, which are essentially watered-down versions of the original that you pay the same price for, sometimes with a sweetener such as sucralose thrown in to fool your taste buds.

Diet soda and these "health" drinks are still a part of the global industrial food chain, requiring all that energy to bring to you, and you get little or *no* nutrition or energy in return. And remember that you can easily obtain the small smattering of vitamins any of these might provide by instead eating whole foods, taking your multivitamin, or having some whole grain breakfast cereal. So can the soda. And remember, zero calories doesn't mean zero impact.

GREEN BENEFITS

A 12-ounce aluminum can is derived from metals mined halfway across the globe. The can itself, in fact, requires 1,643 kilocalories of fossil fuel energy to make, which is usually more than 10 times the food energy that's contained in it (food energy, by the way, in the form of high-fructose corn syrup—nasty). Fill the can with diet soda

SKIP THE ARTIFICIAL SWEETENERS
TO BE LEAN AND GREEN

I have changed my opinion of artificial sweeteners over the years I've been a dietitian. (Full disclosure, I once did some media work for aspartame, but withdrew after I realized that as I personally didn't use it or give it to my children, I could not endorse its use, or the use of any other artificial sweetener for that matter.) Artificial sweeteners are not part of a lean and green lifestyle because they are industrial ingredients; they are often found in industrial foods; they keep your palate focused on sweet foods and beverages; and they don't appear to provide a real advantage to weight loss (there is certainly much data that has found weight loss benefits of several artificial sweeteners, but these studies have subjects on a calorie-controlled diet that includes some artificially sweetened products; of course people are likely to lose weight when following a reduced-calorie plan).

"Artificial sweeteners may give you the illusion of doing something useful to avoid sugars and control your calorie intake," writes Marion Nestle in *What to Eat*, "but it does not take much food to make up for the calories you save, and the sweeteners do not help with what really matters in weight control: eating less and being more active." Exactly. Avoid them.

instead of regular, and you've just spent more than 1,600 fossil fuel calories to bring you precisely zero.[14] Zilch. Totally wasteful.

And though recycling just one aluminum beverage can saves enough electricity to power your TV for 3 hours, we can't just "recycle away" the consequences of our soda habit; recycling still requires energy and water resources. Then there's the teensie inconvenient fact that about $2 billion in recyclable aluminum beverage cans is tossed into landfills every year.[15] It's still taking from the system, using energy and gobbling resources. And if all that is happening just so you can "have your cake and eat it too" by sipping sweet soda without any caloric consequences, consider the size of your own carbon footprint to be a lot bigger than it should be. So take less—and start looking better, saving money, lightening your carbon footprint, and feeling more beautylicious because you know you're doing right by yourself and the planet. In my experience, I have found that people often simply start feeling a lot better once they can the soda completely, even the diet stuff.

In the end, it's pretty simple and straightforward, and deep down you probably know that you should be drinking less anyway. So stay focused on the benefits of greening your glass. It will go a long way toward simplifying your shopping trips; it will save your back from lugging all those liquids into your pantry; it will help rebalance your palate away from the constant craving for sweetness; and it will trim unwanted carbon and pounds from your life.

TAKE ACTION NOW

- When you do splurge on sodas, look for a locally made brand with clean ingredients. Buy in bulk and recycle every stitch of packaging.

- Choose fountain drinks rather than single-serving bottles.

- Choose glass over aluminum cans because they're about twice as energy efficient to produce.

- Make a DIY soda/seltzer at home. You can save money and carbon by investing in a home soda-making machine. (But you won't save any calories.)

- If you absolutely must flavor your beverage, buy the concentrated packets and add them to your own water. Not only is it more cost effective, but you'll also be saving the carbon cost of shipping all that liquid volume.

Perhaps nowhere in the grocery aisles is it as clear just how troubled our calorie intake has become. Perhaps in no area of our diets is it as hard to ignore the clear intersection of weight and warming problems caused by the daily habits of the American consumer. Thank goodness that the way out of both is clear and straightforward. Your own best defense against belly bloat, and Earth's best defense against frivolous waste and carbon burn, are one and the same: sip sustainably.

See? I told you it was easy.

Have you saved room for dessert? Good. Now let's get talking about those green treats.

CHAPTER 14

COFFEE, TEA, AND CHOCOLATE

Why Making These Splurges Sustainable Matters More Than Ever

"For the first time in human history, 'more' is no longer synonymous with 'better.'"

—Bill McKibben, author, *Deep Economy*

YOUR LEAN AND GREEN PRESCRIPTION

ENJOY

Unlimited filtered or purified tap water daily

Fresh brewed coffee or tea (especially green, black, or herbal), regular or decaf, daily, in the amount that you prefer

Up to 1 ounce high-quality dark chocolate (containing at least 60 percent cocoa) 3 or 4 times a week, counted as part of your Sustainable Snacks Prescription

Greener: Tea bags or loose-leaf tea with an eco-chic label

Eco-chic coffee, organic and sustainably produced chocolate

LIMIT

Coffeehouse drinks in a to-go cup

All the "add-ons" (milk, sugar, pumps, whips, etc.)

AVOID

Bottled or canned coffee or tea drinks, especially sweetened ones

Milk chocolate and white chocolate

Chocolate candy, commercial chocolate bars, and other chocolate food products

Coffee. Tea. Chocolate. (Just typing these words heightens my desire to zip down to my "secret stash" for a piece of dark chocolate, despite it being only 8:30 a.m.) Three delicious indulgences that awaken, nourish, comfort, and sustain us.

Coffee and tea are some of civilization's oldest global beverages, and a walk through the brew aisle can read like an exotic novel. They awaken the senses, they awaken the sipper, and because they are plant foods, they deliver several powerful compounds for health.

I'll break down the health benefits of coffee, tea, and chocolate individually for you, but then I think it will be best to talk about the green benefits of all three at once. Why am I considering them together? Because of where they're grown and how they're produced, they are also three foods with many similar issues when it comes to their carbon footprints. And choosing the right kinds matters more than you think. A lot more.

At the end of the chapter, we'll finish on a sweet note by circling back around to tackle the sugars and sweet treats we first addressed in your quick fixes, so you can see how to enjoy these foods on occasion while still staying a beautiful shade of green, and building on all of your successes you've achieved in each chapter.

Coffee's Many Perks

If you happen to be enjoying a cup of coffee while reading this, then sip away without guilt and read on. While coffee has been accused of contributing to a host of ills, including infertility, miscarriage, cancer, and heart disease, this is more a cup of confusion than facts. Actually, the vast body of research seems to point in the other direction—that the health benefits far outweigh the risks.

The past few decades have produced some 19,000 studies examining coffee's impact on health, and, notes health writer Sid Kircheimer, "for the most part, their results are as pleasing as a gulp of freshly brewed Breakfast Blend for the 108 million Americans who routinely enjoy this morning, and increasingly day-long, ritual."[1] In fact, if some pharmaceutical company had invented it as a drug and held a patent, their savvy marketing folks would probably put a spin on coffee that might sound something like this:

"A revolutionary breakthrough drug that boosts mood and enhances performance, can cut your risk of Parkinson's disease and liver cancer by 80 percent, reduce your risk of gallstones by

50 percent, alleviate headaches and asthma, and help protect you from the biggest scourge of American life in the 21st century— type 2 diabetes—all in a safe and delicious package."[2]

And would it surprise you to know that if they said all this, their claims would actually be firmly planted in the research? Let's review the highlights.

LEAN BENEFITS

In addition to being a zero-calorie beverage (and as we just covered in the last chapter, drinking zero calories is a prime strategy for getting lean), coffee is loaded with compounds called quinines that may help improve insulin sensitivity. Other components in coffee have also been shown to improve insulin sensitivity as well as glucose metabolism. These components, namely chlorogenic acid and tocopherols, may explain why coffee drinking helps protect against type 2 diabetes. Coffee also contains magnesium, an important mineral that helps keep your cardiovascular system healthy. And a 2008 study in the *Journal of Agricultural and Food Chemistry* found that the very aroma of coffee triggers relaxation in the brain and activates genes that promote antioxidant activity.[3]

Of course, the oodles of caffeine that come in a triple shot of espresso may be too much of a jolt for many of us. High caffeine intake may send your insulin levels plummeting a couple of hours later, leaving you feeling shaky and looking for refined carbs or sugars to pick you up (aka coffeehouse cravings). And our growing cup sizes can make matters worse if you're sensitive; just rummage through your parents' collection of coffee cups (which, if it's like my parents' collection, contains some lovely specimens from the 1970s) if you want a reminder of just how big our beverages have become in the past 2 decades.

If you decide to purge caffeine from your diet altogether, by all means feel free to do so. You may find you feel much better and ultimately more energized. However, you may also find that this turns you into a crankypants who's no fun to be around until noon. If there's one thing I've learned from the thousands of clients I've talked with, it's woe to the person who stands between a man (or woman) and his caffeine. If that's the case, drink your coffee and don't lose sleep over it. The evidence seems to be on your side that moderate amounts are a safe and tasty addition to a healthy diet. And since you've now purged many other dirty beverages from your diet, coffee may add a delicious variation.

"Moderate coffee consumption" is loosely defined as about 300 milligrams of caffeine a day (two to three cups, depending on the size). However, I find that people have a very broad range of what works and doesn't work for them. Hormonal changes can also affect your tolerance level, so what may have been okay when you were 25 may no longer be the case at age 45. Find your own "best level," and stick to decaf or avoid coffee altogether if that level is zero.

THE CAFFEINE COUNTER[4]

ITEM	CAFFEINE (MG)	ITEM	CAFFEINE (MG)
Brewed coffee, drip (8 oz)	56–120	Dark chocolate (1 oz)	5–35
Espresso (1 oz)	30–50	Soft drink (8 oz)	20–40
Black tea	40–60		

Far worse to your waistline than the coffee itself are those lovely little extras: the full-fat milk, syrups, whipped cream, caramel, and other stuff you are pouring into it. These pack on the pounds, can spike your blood sugar, and can trigger cravings. Check out the calorie counts in the table on the next page to see the cost of your coffee addictions. This information probably isn't a shocker, but as a nutritionist, of course I need to point it out. In addition to hiking up the calories, all these add-ons also obviously hike up the carbon count.

If you do indulge, count any milk that you use in your coffee as part of your 1 cup per day max (from your Dairy Prescription), and count each teaspoon of cream or fat as part of your 6 daily teaspoons (from your Fat Prescription). And try to minimize added sugars as much as possible. For most people, it takes about a week for your taste buds to make the switch to a healthier, leaner brew. If you followed the initial quick fixes in Chapter 3, then chances are you have discovered, as most people do, that you have either adjusted to sugarless coffee and don't crave adding it back, or else you can now add less and can still be satisfied with much smaller amounts. Congratulations, your palate is coming down off the sugar rush!

DOES YOUR COFFEE HAVE MORE CALORIES THAN A CRULLER?[5]

ITEM	CALORIES	ITEM	CALORIES
2 Tbsp whipped cream	15	2 Tbsp nonfat milk	10
2 Tbsp heavy cream	104	1 tsp sugar (white or raw)	16
2 Tbsp half and half	39	1 pump flavored syrup	20
2 Tbsp 2% milk	15		

Green (and Black) Tea

Moving from a highly sugary/milky breakfast mug of coffee to a cup of steaming tea is one of the fastest ways to cut some calories and add some powerful antioxidants to your diet. And many people who are sensitive to coffee may find tea a much better fit for them.

Because tea is composed of plant leaves, it is packed with flavonoids, antioxidants that cut inflammation, improve blood vessel function, and reduce the risk of heart attacks and stroke. Flavonoids also protect against cancer because they fight free radicals and keep carcinogens from wreaking havoc on your cells' DNA.[6]

WILL CAFFEINE HELP ME LOSE WEIGHT?

The caffeine in regular coffee and tea may give you a small additional weight loss advantage, and here's why: A handful of studies on caffeine seem to indicate that people who consume caffeine, eat a low-fat diet, and exercise may experience a small advantage in weight loss (but then again, so will people who combine a low-fat diet with exercise without the caffeine). Caffeine can also act as a mild appetite suppressant, and it stimulates thermogenesis, a metabolic boost through which your body generates heat and energy.

The other reason a bit of caffeine may help you lose weight is that caffeine, in small amounts, can enhance athletic performance (which is one of the reasons it's banned in large doses by the International Olympic Committee). In theory, this means that you can have more effective workouts that burn more calories, helping you lose a bit more weight if your calorie intake remains the same. All of these reasons explain why you often see caffeine listed as an ingredient in diet pills and weight loss supplements (this, plus the fact that caffeine can act as a diuretic, creating very short-term weight loss that is "water weight"—not something I am promoting at all).

My advice? Think of caffeine's benefits as a small plus rather than something that will result in significant weight loss. In some people, caffeine seems to trigger sweet cravings or insulin sensitivity; if this is the case for you, you may want to limit or eliminate caffeine altogether. And I definitely do not suggest you start consuming high levels of caffeine to pump up the weight loss; caffeine triggers your body's "stress response" by elevating the stress hormone cortisol, and too much can cause irritability, stomach upset, and nervousness; increase your heart rate and blood pressure; and interfere with healthy sleep patterns.

LEAN BENEFITS

Want some other reasons to steep yourself in the delicious, slimming power of tea? Other compounds in tea called catechins may give you a little extra weight loss boost. Several studies have found that catechins may help lower body fat mass, waist circumference, body mass index (BMI), and LDL cholesterol.[7] (As with caffeine, this explains why tea is a popular addition these days, being added to products from energy bars to supplements to breakfast cereals.)

Green and black tea may even offer benefits in addition to the catechins. The natural plant compounds in these teas (which are both from the *Camellia sinensis* plant) help fight cancer, oxidative cell damage, infection, and even fat metabolism. New research suggests that tea may help fight osteoporosis and stabilize blood sugar levels.[8]

So find a way to start including tea regularly. I recommend that you include a cup of tea in the afternoon daily; if you're an afternoon coffee or diet soda drinker (and if you were, I'm gonna assume that was the *old* you and not the *new* you), this is a great place to make the move to green tea for a mild caffeine boost that's sweeter to your health and the planet. It helps give you an afternoon ritual without the calories. And it can be gentler to your stomach than simply another cup of coffee. Try to find a store near you that carries some high-quality loose-leaf tea, or order some online (they're such a far cry from the droopy tea bags of your grandparents' generation, and their exotic scents are the next best thing to time travel). There are several great national brands, such as Tazo and Numi, that offer high-quality teas in easy-to-use, ecofriendly boxes. Plus, you may be surprised to learn that even global brands such as Lipton are moving toward "sustainable teas." In fact, by 2015 Lipton aims to be the largest brand in the world certified sustainable by the Rainforest Action Network, and I expect this will be at a super-affordable price. So find what works best for you to jump-start your way to a leaner, greener drinking habit.

Chocolate

When I announced I wanted to become a dietitian, my mother had but one thing to say:

"Please," she begged, "find some reason why I should be eating more chocolate!"

Well, Mom, I've got sweet news for you.

Chocolate has long been revered for its rich flavor and aphrodisiac qualities. The Aztecs believed that chocolate was a gift from the gods. The early Spanish explorers introduced chocolate to Europe in

1520, where it quickly became reserved for the nobility. And thanks to what experts call its hedonic appeal (that magical elixir of fat, sugar, texture, and aroma), it easily claims the title "Most Commonly Craved Food in North America."[9] So once again, my mom is in good company, I guess.

But high-quality dark chocolate is more than simply tantalizing to the taste buds. It is filled with bioactive compounds that have been shown to help keep you healthy, including flavonoids that can significantly improve your arteries' endothelial function, lower blood pressure (BP), and increase bloodflow to the brain.[10] A 2007 study found that one small square of dark chocolate a day lowered BP by a few points and kept it there; this is a big deal, because in BP, an improvement of just a few points can cut your risk of stroke or heart attack.[11] Dark chocolate is also high in antioxidants called proanthocyanins that mop up free radicals. And cocoa, like coffee, is rich in magnesium, another important mineral in cardiovascular health. Because chocolate, like coffee and tea, comes from a plant, it shouldn't surprise you that, like other plant foods, it is teeming with compounds that promote health at the deepest levels.

LEAN BENEFITS

Now when it comes to the lean benefits, let's be honest. Endorsing chocolate as a nutritionist is a slippery slope. This category gets ugly fast. Those candy bars in your local supermarket that are loaded with extra sugars, hydrogenated oils, waxes, and chemicals are *not* in your Prescription. So there are a few big qualifications I'd like to make in order to make sure this Prescription helps get you to your lean goals instead of right back into your fat pants.

- Buy only really good quality dark chocolate, labeled as containing at least 60 percent cocoa.
- This is one area of your diet where buying in bulk may backfire, big time. If you have to buy single servings to keep a handle on portions, then do so. It's a wise investment.
- To help be sure you keep it at 1 ounce, eat your prescription only *after* a meal, when you're already satisfied and feeling

full. Hitting the chocolate drawer at 10:30 a.m. when you're hungry "in the name of health" is a recipe for disaster.

- If chocolate is a trigger food for you, or you have serious problems with portion control, avoid this Prescription altogether.

The real health benefits of dark chocolate come from the flavonoids in the cocoa plant itself; the more that cocoa is processed, the more these powerful flavonoids are lost. Many commercial chocolates remove these flavonols because of the bitter or astringent flavor notes they can offer. But many people (and I bet you will, too) find that the taste of high-quality dark chocolate is heavenly good, much more interesting than the bland, super-sweet commercial stuff. Some dark chocolate offers the same level of complexity as a fine wine, which makes it easier to be satisfied with less. By the way, it goes pretty well *with* your wine, too.

Dark chocolate also makes an amazing pairing with dried fruit. When I was meeting with publishers trying to sell this book idea, it was November 2007. I brought in my "green treats"—a 1-ounce mix of sustainable dark chocolate and dried Utah cherries—an antioxidant- and flavor-rich snack (served in a reusable glass spice jar—a great portion control tool!). People loved it. And you will, too. Here are some other fun ways I personally like to use my splurge.

GREEN TREAT #1

Pack 1 ounce dark chocolate pieces and 1 ounce walnuts, almonds, or locally dried fruit (I use cherries, but use whatever's in your area) in a reusable snack container (e.g., an empty spice jar) and bring to work. Savor in front of jealous colleagues.

GREEN TREAT #2

Melt 1 ounce dark chocolate and dip ½ cup fresh fruit in season (such as berries, citrus wedges, cherries, or pear slices) in it. Smile. Repeat.

GREEN TREAT #3

Enjoy those last two sips from your daily dose of red wine with 1 ounce of dark chocolate after a meal. Combine all ingredients in your mouth. Swirl, savor, and then swallow.

So remember, a little goes a long way—both in calories and in health benefits. The two keys are high quality and small portions. Quality over quantity. The rewards to your taste buds and body will be tremendous.

GREEN BENEFITS

So now to the green benefits of our three indulgences. What do chocolate, coffee, and tea all have in common? A deep connection to the vital "carbon sink" of Planet Earth—the rainforest.

The rainforest is a new but significant element to your food's carbon footprint that we haven't yet touched upon anywhere else. Every single American has a huge stake in protecting it, and here's why: Tropical forests literally act like lungs for the Earth, helping to slow global warming. The rainforest, aside from just being a nice "science unit" for school kids, provides one of the few counterweights to our SUV lifestyle—and our SUV diet. So much so, in fact, that the international community soon may be compensating countries such as Brazil for keeping it intact rather than clearing it for Western-style growth and development.

If you are an average American, the rainforest is a lot closer to your pantry than you may even realize. You see, agriculture is the number-one cause of rainforest destruction worldwide. What does that rather dry-sounding fact have to do with you? Much of it is being done in order to feed Americans cheaply and efficiently. How? Fast-food hamburgers. Inexpensive chocolate products. Bargain-priced OJ. And cheap soybean and palm oil (being driven by leading US agribusiness companies) to serve as cheap ingredients in our industrial food chain.[12] These are just four examples. Purchasing rainforest products (or products grown in areas where rainforest used to be) will influence your own carbon footprint significantly.

According to the United Nations Environment Program, tropical deforestation is responsible for about 20 percent of total annual global warming emissions. When the trees are cleared, we not only lose their ability to offset carbon dioxide, but also the harvest process itself creates a carbon impact. This makes tropical deforestation second behind fossil fuels in terms of climate impact. Because of this very real "double warming" effect, you can see how these foods can significantly impact the size of your own carbon feet.

When it comes to coffee, tea, chocolate, and spices, even in their greener shades, there are several carbon elements to consider.

- They are grown in exotic locations (read: the developing world with varying degrees of regulation, oversight, and accountability).

- They are inherently more processed products. You're not simply picking off a vine or plucking out of the ground. Just to become a basic "staple," these foods typically require sorting, roasting, and grinding to become edible.

- They must be transported from that exotic location, often passing through many hands, which means many steps, which typically packs on the carbon.

Even the great companies doing organic and sustainable work (and there are many) still have to contend with these core issues. This is to say nothing of the companies who then take these staples and layer pounds of petroleum onto them by transforming them into things such as fluffy candy bars, microwaveable hot fudge sauces, coffee-flavored creamers, and breakfast bars with green tea extract.

David Pimentel, PhD, from Cornell University, considered one of the pioneers of "food energy" research, shows you why pound for pound these are some of the more energy-intensive foods to bring to you. (I've included some other foods we've also covered to give you some basis of comparison.)

Yikes! Aren't these total carbon belchers to the planet? Why aren't you calling this a Hummer, the way you've already panned my steak? If this is what you're thinking, I don't blame you, but read on and I'll explain.

Here's why the splurge is worth it. The health benefits of the compounds in coffee, tea, and chocolate are significant and real, just as real, in fact, as the health *drawbacks* that come with eating too much of that steak.

HOW MUCH FOSSIL FUEL IS IN THAT TREAT?[14]

FOOD	CALORIES OF FOSSIL FUEL/KG
Milk	354
Ice cream	880
Baked goods	1,485
Beet sugar	5,660
Breakfast cereals	15,675
Chocolate	18,591
Coffee	18,948

Even more important, these foods present a direct opportunity to use your dollars in a way that encourages preservation of the most vital carbon cooler of all—the rainforest. It's your chance to help leverage American eating habits for something good in the fight against global warming—to keep the rainforest alive rather than burning it down to make room for those cattle that will end up in your quarter-pounder that costs you less than a buck. Or for coffee that's a bit cheaper. In other words, by choosing organic and sustainable choices when it comes to coffee, tea, and chocolate, you will actually help preserve this critical resource that is counteracting your own high-carbon lifestyle. (Your other Lean and Green Prescriptions throughout this book will also help keep you out of the rainforest.)

Think your teensie contributions won't really matter when compared to, say, the future automobile growth of India? Think again. Consider that if just one US household switches to coffee that protects bird habitat (look for labels that include the words "Rainforest Alliance," "Bird Friendly," or "Shade Grown"), the annual savings can protect more than 9,000 square feet of rainforest. If the population of Seattle practiced this, a rainforest the size of Seattle could be spared every year.[15]

Small, daily choices matter. In fact, the current state of your health and energy (or lack thereof) at this very moment is in large part a sum of those daily choices that you have made in the past. It's not too late to begin rewriting your future.

Finally, let's talk a moment about the cost of choosing organic and sustainable products over cheaper substitutes. After all, I can hear people's reaction to this chapter: *"But organic coffee and chocolate costs a lot more!"*

Here's the deal: If you started this program with the eating habits of an average American, you have already freed up significant money by purging many high-carbon (which often means higher-cost) foods from your diet. I've tried to pack this book with tons of tips for realigning your food budget so as to be lean and green without spending any extra money. And those tips even come into play here: Eating less of the high-quality chocolate and making

THE "HAMBURGERIZATION" OF THE RAINFOREST[16]

The United States imports roughly 100,000,000 pounds of beef from Central America each year. Once this beef passes US inspection, there are no "country of origin" labels (as there are with seafood) to let you know where it came from, so it's hard to know. But this beef may be in your fast-food burger, or it may end up in processed foods such as frozen dinners, chilis, stews, and pet food.

What is the exact carbon footprint of chopping down a carbon cooler to make room for grazing cattle? Here are some fun stats to keep in mind next time you're tempted to think your choices don't really matter.

The amount of rainforest destroyed for each quarter-pound burger that comes from Brazil[17]	55 square feet
Amount of carbon released in 1 day by driving a typical American car	3 kilograms
Amount of carbon released by clearing enough Costa Rican rainforest to produce beef for one hamburger	75 kilograms
Length of time before the Indonesian forests would be completely gone if they were cleared to produce enough beef for Indonesians to eat as much beef, per person, as the people of the United States do	3.5 years
Length of time before the Costa Rican rainforest would be completely gone if it were cleared to produce enough beef for Costa Ricans to eat as much beef, per person, as the people of the United States do	1 year

your coffee at home rather than buying it from a doughnut shop are two quick examples.

But let's be frank for a moment about those household expenses that are outside of your grocery bill. Even in our depressed economy, there are still a few places to "find" a few extra bucks. I know this from personal experience, as my own family has weathered financial ups and downs of job changes, starting a business, and disability.

Be satisfied with your current iPod playlist. Cancel the TiVo or the 600 channels. Skip that mall pretzel or iced tea. Acknowledge your love affair with shoes, even bargain-priced shoes. Give coupons for time and love for birthdays and holidays rather than a costly present. Or skip just one "coffeehouse" purchase a week and free up about $16 a month to put toward higher-level products. Or whatever works for you; most of the good money management books are chock-full of ideas for "finding money" (in fact, I believe one even dubbed it "the Latte Factor"). Even when money seems tight, chances are, it may be an easy excuse for something else that's holding you back. "I really don't want to do this; it seems hard; it's different; I don't want to change; I like being able to have (insert vice here)." If that's the case, please turn directly to Chapter 15.

TAKE ACTION NOW

Shop for eco-chic labels. Especially in this category of foods, the power of eco-chic labels runs a lot deeper than just looking fashionable. It is truly connected to the well-being of the ecosystems that can help slow global warming. Rainforest Alliance Certified programs are in place for coffee, tea, cocoa, citrus, and bananas. Sustainably harvested, bird-friendly, and organic are also great options. Even for tea, coffee, and other items produced in non-rainforest zones (such as parts of Africa), you can still be a strong force shaping the environment. Because soy and palm plantations are a significant source of rainforest destruction, too, ideally, expand this to include any foods with soy or palm ingredients as well.

Buy "green" bananas. Fifteen percent of all bananas in the international trade carry the Rainforest Alliance Certification. Ask your supermarket to carry them if they don't already (Chiquita is one of the largest companies with this certification). And my personal tip? Save bananas for the dead of winter when you may have little else available; fill your cart with local seasonal produce as much as your growing season allows.

Check the zip code of that OJ. Many brands of orange juice sold in the United States are made from oranges that come from Central or South America, which means they've likely been grown

YOUR GUIDE TO THE ECO LABELS

Here's a quick rundown of what is the minimum requirement in order to make each claim. Some are more rigorous than others, and some deal with social versus environmental issues, so read carefully.[18]

BIRD FRIENDLY
■ Coffee is grown under conditions that support healthy bird habitats.

■ Coffee is grown under a tree canopy with a minimum of 40 percent shade.

■ Coffee is grown organically, according to USDA organic standards.

RAINFOREST ALLIANCE
■ Crops are grown using integrated pest management systems that limit the use of agrochemicals.

■ Crops are grown using measures that conserve water, soil, and wildlife habitat.

■ Farm laborers are paid salaries and benefits equal to or greater than the legal minimum wage of their countries.

SHADE GROWN
This is the loosest regulation of all, so be savvy. Look for clearly defined minimum shade coverage requirements and third-party certification. The Bird Friendly certification is currently the most rigorous. Protects bird habitat.

FAIR TRADE CERTIFIED
■ Farmers and workers are guaranteed a minimum price of $1.26 per pound ($1.41 per pound if organic), which is higher than average market rates, for their product.*

■ Trade is conducted directly between farmer-owned cooperatives and buyers.

■ Crops are grown using soil and water conservation measures that restrict the use of agrochemicals.

For a list of companies that carry Fair Trade coffee, visit the Web site of TransFair USA, the US fair trade labeling organization (www.transfairusa.org).

*Since growers receive a minimum price regardless of what you pay for a Fair Trade Certified product, you can shop around to find the lowest retail price.

USDA CERTIFIED ORGANIC
■ Farmers emphasize the use of renewable resources and the conservation of soil and water to enhance environmental quality.

■ Crops are grown without using synthetic fertilizer or the most persistent pesticides.

■ Crops are produced without genetic engineering or ionizing radiation.

■ Crops are processed and handled separately from conventional coffee.

on land that was once rainforest. If it comes from South of the Border, absolutely choose an eco-chic label.

Set a greener tea time. Choose tea bags, packets, and pouches over tea that's already bottled. Bottled teas often don't have the same levels of powerful antioxidant capacity as teas that you steep yourself; they can contain sweeteners (and thus empty calories); and they're much heavier to transport per serving than just the tea. Plus, of course, you have all the added packaging and the higher cost per serving.

Spice it up smartly. Staples like cinnamon, vanilla, ginger, black pepper, cayenne, and paprika typically come from tropical forests. If you're on a limited budget, pick the three you use the most and switch to sustainable brands of those.

Go for green treats. Buying nuts, fruit, and chocolate that are sustainably harvested helps keep the forests and the economies that depend on them economically viable and intact. It also helps ensure that the type of business being done overseas isn't completely undoing the "carbon savings" you've just congratulated yourself on by installing LED lights back home.

In today's brightly lit, sterile supermarket environment, it is easy to lose sight of these deeper connections that run between exotic ingredients and their magnified impact on global warming. Our choices at the coffee counter, the chocolate aisle, the banana bin, or the burger joint linger for much longer than just on our lips, or even our hips. They reverberate across the planet, drawing in other lives, communities, and ecosystems halfway across the globe. In fact, perhaps in no other part of our diets is the "ripple effect" of our choices truly as global as these parts of our pantries and our lives.

So wake up and smell the coffee, the green coffee.

As celebrated chef Deborah Madison wrote, "It is impossible to take up the subject of food without thinking about everything else that it touches, which is, in the end, life itself."[19] Awaken to these connections.

Awaken to them and let them inspire you to take action.

MY TOP TIPS FOR LEAN AND GREEN SWEET TREATS

Obviously, life is just sweeter with the occasional treat. Learning how to enjoy them without sabotaging your commitment to healthy eating is the key to lasting success, so here are your guidelines as you move into the maintenance phase of your program. How do you do it? Here's how.

Keep it occasional. Really occasional—at most, a couple of times a month. Here's a basic fact: The more regularly you indulge, the more likely you are to gain weight. You'll also start to retrain your palate to crave sugar if you eat sweets too often. The Go Green Get Lean Diet is designed to provide about 1,600 calories a day, including meals and snacks. In order to continue to lose weight (or to maintain the weight you've lost on this program), it is important that you don't start eating more calories.

I have tried to provide some sweeter options on your sustainable snacks list, including chocolate, to help you work in sweeter calories on occasion. But for those moments when you *do* feel like indulging . . .

Keep it small. "Right foods, right portions" applies here too. Something that fits in the palm of your hand is a good rule of thumb (specifically, that is about a 2- by 2-inch square, or no more than ½ cup). Serve with a heaping side of fresh, seasonal fruit if you want more volume.

Keep it clean. Don't waste calories on subpar food; insist on high-quality ingredients, and you'll get the highest level of taste and satisfaction. Use all that you've learned in your 6-week program to choose sweet treats made with clean ingredient lists: clean fats, dark chocolate, organic local butter, fruits and nuts, and none of the additives or preservatives of industrial food.

Make it fit. If you do enjoy a sweet but want to keep your calories within the 1,600 range, here are some tips: Skip the wine, exercise an extra 30 minutes, or enjoy two of the lower-calorie sustainable snacks to make room for the splurge. And just like with chocolate, don't eat your sweet treat on an empty stomach—that's a recipe for disaster. Instead, enjoy it after a meal; you'll be satisfied with much less.

Know thyself. If sweets are a trigger food for you, or you have trouble managing portions, I highly recommend that you omit them altogether (and think in terms of yearly rather than monthly splurges), or seek the professional counsel of a registered dietitian.

PART VI

TREADING MORE LIGHTLY—FOREVER

CHAPTER 15

STEP INTO MY OFFICE: YOUR PERSONAL PEP TALK

66We are the first generation of Americans in the Energy-Climate Era. This is not about the whales anymore. It is about us. And what we do about the challenges of energy and climate, conservation and preservation, will tell our kids who we really are.99

. —Thomas L. Friedman, *Hot, Flat, and Crowded*

We are standing literally at a crossroads, facing some of the most significant and far-reaching choices we have yet had to make. In ways few of us probably ever thought of before, we are now seeing that our own personal health is deeply intertwined with the health of the planet.

It is time to face your life. Literally. To recognize that at perhaps no other time has it been more true to say "you are what you eat." The question is, What are you consuming?

The follow-up question is, Now knowing this, do you simply do nothing, or do you take the steps needed to chart a new course, one that is healthier for you and the planet?

The power of diet is stronger than any single drug to create better health within yourself. Everything in our diet works together to create health or disease. And it can start working fast to heal and cleanse your body. Further, it is these same chronic, daily choices that affect your personal carbon footprint that you are leaving in the world.

While it's easy to pass the responsibility on to our government or point fingers at the rapid industrialization of China or countless other players, the fact is as an American, each of us needs to accept the consequences that our food choices are having on the rest of the planet. Myself included, your vegan coworker who bikes to work, your next-door neighbor who has six kids and two SUVs, and *you*. We are all in this together. It is not about perfection, it is not about becoming a self-sufficient hermit and subsisting on a pleasureless diet, but it is about taking personal responsibility for our health and our personal role in the global warming crisis and committing to a new era of stewardship for our own bodies and the planet.

Only you can change your diet. Yes, you have your nutritionist (me), your friends and family, and possibly your children to look to for inspiration, and together all of these people can help you do great things and create tremendous momentum and change. This book has given you your blueprint to succeed, but at the end of the day, it's up to you. Not your friends, not your spouse, but *you.*

But let me assure you: You *can* change your life. I have seen it happen hundreds of times. The pride, satisfaction, and deep joy that come from working to reshape your habits are gold. The lean new you, and the pride in knowing you've cut your carbon footprint, are merely the icing on a delicious and sustainable cake.

Yes, you are what you eat. But you are also what you *think.* You can sharpen your focus in an instant on either the positives or the negatives, and here's a secret: The people who fail do so because they focus on the negatives. Their brains start clinging to all they *won't* be having and eating; they focus on their deprivation if they change their eating habits. In fact, their brains are so panicked and churning with their old paradigms and old "internal monologues" (the stories we all tell about ourselves when it comes to our identities and our weight) that they have no room for their *possibilities*—all of the incredible things they can become if they make the room for it and begin a new, fresh, tasty, and lean story.

So make room for your potential. Let go of whatever part of your past is holding you back. Clear away the excessive noise from overwhelming choice and mega portions, and let your possibilities start to speak to you in that silent space. Bring your impact as an American into sharper focus. Americans are using a whopping 25 percent of the world's resources—living high on the hog in every sense—despite being about 5 percent of the total people on the planet. We need to step up. Take control. Your food choices come with three costs—to your health, to your wallet, and to the planet. And the next meal offers an opportunity to begin to heal.

The people who tell themselves positive, energizing, uplifting stories are the ones who succeed. Those who wallow in the past, the negatives, and self-pity get only one place: nowhere. I have seen this with my clients many times; what one client defines as "hard, difficult, expensive, and depriving" another client defines as "exciting, life-changing, and energizing." Guess who succeeds in a fantastic way? Guess who fails miserably? You guessed it. You create your own reality in your mind.

So tape up a picture of some fabulously healthy-looking lean person, or put up a picture of your kids or grandkids, or your favorite quotation that taps deep into your own power to change and become inspired. Toss out the gossip mags and replace them with a *National Geographic* that has a picture of a polar bear clinging to an ice floe on the cover. Remind yourself why this matters to you. To your children. To the world. And that you can do it.

Yes, you *can* shed your old thought patterns and habits that aren't working for you, that weigh down your mind and cause you to eat and weigh down your body. I promise you it is possible. All you have to do is begin to think past the next 5 minutes; replace your old thinking with a healthier, truer, deeper thinking that extends into the next days, weeks, months, and years. You can replace it with a new way of acting, thinking, and being. You can become lighter, cleaner, clearer in purpose and action. As is written in Psalm 139: *You are wonderfully and fearfully made.* Tap into that wonder. You will be amazed to find that it can work wonders.

What's at stake? *You* lie in the balance—your health, your weight, your struggle to look and feel the best you can. Your *family* lies in the balance. And now it's become clear that this *planet,* too, lies in the balance. The question is, Do you think those things are worth fighting for?

While there will continue to be a steady march of newer, "revolutionary" approaches for both the health care and the global warming crisis, there is an older, simple, less expensive, immediate truth as well, one that has become increasingly hard for Americans to hear with the ever-growing drone of their blindingly fast, resource-heavy, overscheduled, overconsumptive lifestyles:

Buy less.

Consume less.

Eat clean.

Drink clean.

Think more.

Move more.

Live simply.

Indeed, many of history's greatest religious leaders have embraced these very tenets, and while we're in a vastly different context of time and place, it seems to ring as true today as ever when it comes to the health of our world.

The question is, Can we clean up our act? I believe you can.

Do you have what it takes to reach your greatest potential? To tap into your immense power as a consumer, to take responsibility for the cost of your food choices to yourself, to your children, and to humanity? I believe that you do. And I think that in your newfound silence, you believe it, too.

The stakes have never been higher. The Earth, your health, and the health of your children lie in the balance.

Now, let's eat.

CHAPTER 16

4 WEEKS OF SEASONAL EATING AND RECIPES

Spring Menu

SOUP OF THE WEEK: Minty Spinach Pea Soup

PASTA OF THE WEEK: Spring Orzo Pasta with Edamame

As your own herbs come up this season, chop and add them into your salad dressings, on top of eggs, onto spring vegetables, or anywhere you like. They not only provide flavor but often provide powerful healing plant compounds.

Be sure to enjoy two sustainable snacks (page 40) daily.

	BREAKFAST	LUNCH	DINNER
MONDAY	1 cup Warm Barley and Quinoa Porridge (recipe p. 236) with ½ cup Soymilk, 2 Tbsp walnuts, ½ cup fresh cherries, 1 tsp local honey (307 calories)	1½ cups Minty Spinach Pea Soup (recipe p. 238) 1 small whole wheat pita tucked with ⅔ cup Eggless Egg Salad (recipe p. 280) (414 calories)	4 oz grilled wild salmon with ½ cup Rhubarb Compote (recipe p. 249) 1 cup Grilled Asparagus with Lemon (recipe p. 241) 1 cup steamed brown rice (593 calories)
TUESDAY	Poached Egg with ½ cup wilted Spinach (or extra asparagus) (recipe p. 237) ½ whole grain English muffin ½ cup nonfat yogurt with ½ cup strawberries and 2 Tbsp almonds (326 calories)	1 Grilled Veggie Burger in Whole Wheat Pita Pocket with shredded carrot and local lettuce (recipe p. 243) 1 oz dried local cherries or other fruit (410 calories)	1 cup Spring Orzo Pasta with Edamame (recipe p. 244) 2 cups Spring Lettuce Salad with 1 Tbsp Tuscan Lemon Vinaigrette (recipe p. 239) (645 calories)

	BREAKFAST	LUNCH	DINNER
WEDNESDAY	1½ cups Gorgeous Green Smoothie (recipe p. 273) 1 oz almonds (319 calories)	⅔ cup extra Eggless Egg Salad in whole wheat pita with local lettuce greens 1½ cups sliced local apricots and strawberries (434 calories)	1¼ cups Tofu Cashew Stir-Fry with Sugar Snap Peas (recipe p. 245) 1 cup steamed brown rice with spring onions (500 calories)
THURSDAY	2 Tbsp almond butter on 1 slice of whole grain local bread 1 Tbsp extra Rhubarb Compote ½ cup nonfat organic local yogurt with ½ cup fresh cherries (394 calories)	1½ cups extra Minty Spinach Pea Soup 8 whole grain crackers 2 fresh local Apricots Stuffed with 2 tsp local Goat Cheese and drizzled with honey (recipe p. 248) (397 calories)	4 oz Grilled Cajun Shrimp Skewers (US farmed) (recipe p. 247) 1 heaping cup Baby Beets with Orange Zest on spring lettuce (recipe p. 243) ½ cup extra Spring Orzo Pasta with Edamame (514 calories)
FRIDAY	⅔ cup Southwest Tofu Scramble with ⅓ cup black beans and spring onions (recipe p. 237) 1 slice whole grain local bread (327 calories)	1 Hummus Wrap (recipe p. 243) 1 cup fresh sliced apricot and cherries (466 calories)	2 Spicy Tofu Tacos (recipe p. 246) 2 cups Spring Lettuce Salad with 1 Tbsp Tuscan Lemon Vinaigrette (623 calories)
SATURDAY	2 Multigrain Pancakes (recipe p. 236) 2 Tbsp warm Rhubarb Compote 1 soy sausage ½ cup Greek yogurt with ½ cup sliced cherries (394 calories)	1¼ cups extra Tofu Cashew Stir-Fry with Sugar Snap Peas ½ cup Greek yogurt with ½ cup sliced cherries (394 calories)	4 oz Ginger Chicken Kebabs (recipe p. 247) 1 cup Asparagus Salad with Sesame Ginger Vinaigrette (recipe p. 240) 1 cup extra steamed brown rice (571 calories)
SUNDAY	1 cup your favorite whole grain breakfast cereal with ½ cup soymilk 1 sliced apricot 2 Tbsp chopped almonds (274 calories)	4 oz extra Ginger Chicken Kebabs 1½ cups Spring Lettuce Salad with ½ cup beans and 1 Tbsp Sweet Tarragon Dressing (recipe p. 242) (444 calories)	1 Wild Game Burger (or mushroom burger) (recipe p. 248) 1 cup Spinach Salad with ½ cup Strawberries, 1 Tbsp Almonds, and ½ tsp Poppy Seeds (recipe p. 242) (572 calories)

Summer Menu

Summer is the easiest time of all to eat like a locavore and still live like a king. I highly encourage you to substitute local fruit and vegetable choices from your area to the extent possible when available (e.g., huckleberries, or stuffed local peppers instead of tomatoes).

Be sure to enjoy two sustainable snacks (page 40) every day.

	BREAKFAST	LUNCH	DINNER
MONDAY	1½ cups Summer Smoothie (recipe p. 250) 1 oz walnuts (339 calories)	Farm Salad (recipe p. 254) 2 Tbsp Tuscan Lemon Vinaigrette (recipe p. 239) 1 slice crusty whole grain local bread (505 calories)	4 oz grilled green fish with ½ cup Fresh Peach Salsa (recipe p. 254) 1 ear grilled summer corn ¾ cup steamed baby fingerling potatoes (533 calories)
TUESDAY	1 cup Chilled Oatmeal with Summer Fruit (recipe p. 250) drizzle with 2 tsp raw local honey (351 calories)	Open-Faced Turkey Melt (recipe p. 255) 1 cup fresh local blackberries (415 calories)	2 Fresh Corn, Pepper, and Black Bean Tacos (recipe p. 257) 1 cup Easy Gazpacho (recipe p. 252) (615 calories)
WEDNESDAY	2 multigrain waffles 1 soy sausage ½ cup fresh strawberries and blueberries heated with 2 tsp raw local honey (366 calories)	1⅓ cups Easy Gazpacho 1 cup Tabbouleh Salad with White Beans (recipe p. 253) (373 calories)	½ Herbed Zucchini Frittata (recipe p. 251) 1½ cups steamed green beans with garlic 1 slice crusty whole grain local bread ½ cup plum and nectarine slices (528 calories)

	BREAKFAST	LUNCH	DINNER
THURSDAY	½ Herbed Zucchini Frittata 1 cup mixed raspberries and blackberries (352 calories)	2 pieces of Falafel in Pita (recipe p. 250) 2 fresh local plums (372 calories)	2 Stuffed Tomatoes with Quinoa, Raisins, and Mint (recipe p. 256) 1½ cups local green beans sautéed with 1 tsp olive oil, ginger, and garlic 1 ear grilled summer corn (541 calories)
FRIDAY	1 cup nonfat Greek yogurt with 2 Tbsp pistachios 1 tsp raw local honey ⅓ cup local cinnamon granola 1 cup cubed fresh local melon (356 calories)	1 extra Stuffed Tomato 1 slice crusty whole grain local bread Unlimited summer greens and sliced cucumbers tossed with 2 Tbsp Sweet Tarragon Dressing (recipe p. 242) (425 calories)	4 oz grilled green fish with unlimited fresh local dill and green onions 1 cup Tabbouleh Salad with White Beans 2 fresh Grilled Local Plums (recipe p. 258) (534 calories)
SATURDAY	2 Tbsp all-natural peanut butter on 1 slice of whole grain local bread 2 tsp farmers' market jam ½ cup cubed cantaloupe mixed with ½ cup blackberries (369 calories)	Farm Salad with Hard-Boiled Egg (recipe p. 254) ½ cup sliced strawberries with a splash of balsamic vinegar (354 calories)	2 cups Easy Gazpacho 8 Crunchy Herbed Pita Triangles (recipe p. 255) ½ cup Cumin Lime Hummus (recipe p. 254) (574 calories)
SUNDAY	1 cup whole grain breakfast cereal with ½ cup nonfat milk ½ cup fresh raspberries 2 Tbsp chopped walnuts 2 Tbsp sunflower seeds (397 calories)	2 pieces of Falafel in Pita 1 fresh local watermelon slice (350 calories)	4 oz grilled organic local chicken 1 cup Fresh Peach Salsa 1 ear grilled summer corn 1 slice crusty whole grain local bread 1½ cups local green beans with ginger and garlic (555 calories)

Fall Menu

If you have access to a nice local apple cider, consider swapping your other 100 percent juice (if you can afford the extra calories) during the height of cider season.

Be sure to enjoy two sustainable snacks (page 40) every day.

	BREAKFAST	LUNCH	DINNER
MONDAY	Fried Local Egg Open-Faced Sandwich (recipe p. 260) ½ cup nonfat Greek yogurt mixed with 1 chopped local apple (333 calories)	1⅔ cups Autumn Squash and Pinto Bean Chili with Cinnamon and Cumin (recipe p. 263) 1 Hearty Corn Muffin (recipe p. 268) (361 calories)	4 oz grilled green fish with Balsamic Onions (recipe p. 269) ¾ cup steamed purple potatoes ⅔ cup Gorgeous Greens in a Flash (recipe p. 265) (586 calories)
TUESDAY	Cinnamon Granola Parfait with local dried fruit (recipe p. 259) (335 calories)	½ cup Crunchy Curried Chicken Salad with dried cranberries, celery, and almonds in a small whole wheat wrap (recipe p. 264) Late summer peach (443 calories)	½ Fall Green Frittata (recipe p. 261) 1 slice whole grain local bread ⅔ cup Roasted Carrots with Mint (recipe p. 269) (455 calories)
WEDNESDAY	⅔ cup Hot Quinoa Cereal with 1 spiced pear (recipe p. 259) 1 Tbsp chopped walnuts (395 calories)	1⅔ cups extra Autumn Squash and Pinto Bean Chili with Cinnamon and Cumin 1 extra Hearty Corn Muffin (361 calories)	¾ cup Wild Venison Ragù over 1 cup polenta (recipe p. 272) ⅔ cup extra Roasted Carrots with Mint 1¼ cups Buttery Cabbage (recipe p. 271) (571 calories)
THURSDAY	½ extra Fall Green Frittata ¾ cup extra purple potatoes (313 calories)	⅓ cup extra Crunchy Curried Chicken Salad with dried cranberries, celery, and almonds on a slice of toasted local whole grain bread ½ cup fresh local pear slices (358 calories)	½ Wild Rice Stuffed Acorn Squash (recipe p. 267) 1 cup Shaved Fennel Salad (recipe p. 260) (645 calories)

	BREAKFAST	LUNCH	DINNER
FRIDAY	Slice of toasted whole grain local bread 2 Tbsp almond butter 1 tsp honey or maple syrup 4 oz apple cider or ½ cup sliced fall fruit (350 calories)	½ extra Wild Rice Stuffed Acorn Squash 1 fresh local pear (571 calories)	¾ cup extra Wild Venison Ragù over 1 cup polenta 1 cup extra Shaved Fennel Salad (479 calories)
SATURDAY	1 multigrain waffle, topped with frozen local berries, a dollop of plain nonfat local yogurt, and 2 tsp maple syrup 1 spiced pear (378 calories)	½ cup Eggless Egg Salad pita pocket with shredded carrot (recipe p. 280) 2 Tbsp dried local cranberries or cherries (408 calories)	1½ cups Chickpeas and Tofu in Indian Red Sauce (recipe p. 270) 1 cup whole wheat couscous ¾ cup Gorgeous Greens in a Flash (518 calories)
SUNDAY	4 Sweet Potato Pancakes (recipe p. 262) ½ cup Cinnamon Apple Compote (recipe p. 287) 1 soy sausage (402 calories)	1½ cups extra Chickpeas and Tofu in Indian Red Sauce 1 cup whole wheat couscous (405 calories)	4 oz grilled green fish with rub or herbs of your choice ⅔ cup Warmed Beets with Walnut Oil and Chopped Walnuts (recipe p. 266) 1 cup wild rice (502 calories)

Winter Menu

Winter can be a glorious time to eat and still stay in season. If you live in a colder region, this might be your highest carbon eating season the first time around, as you rely a bit more on certain items from neighboring regions. So when summer next rolls around, load up your freezer and pantry with all that your area is overflowing with at the farmers' markets.

Be sure to enjoy two sustainable snacks (page 40) every day.

	BREAKFAST	LUNCH	DINNER
MONDAY	1 slice toasted Pumpkin Cranberry Loaf (recipe p. 274) 1 cup nonfat Greek yogurt with 2 Tbsp chopped nuts (418 calories)	1½ cups Hearty Winter Bean Chili (recipe p. 277) 6 whole grain crackers 1 orange (427 calories)	4 oz Roasted Rosemary Chicken with ¾ cup Roasted Fall Vegetables (recipe p. 286) 1½ cups Chopped Watercress Salad with 1 Tbsp pistachios and 2 tsp Pomegranate Vinaigrette (recipe p. 278) (449 calories)
TUESDAY	1 slice toasted whole grain local bread topped with 2 Tbsp cashew butter and 1 Tbsp Cinnamon Apple Compote (recipe p. 287) ½ grapefruit (340 calories)	Whole wheat wrap with 2 oz diced extra Roasted Rosemary Chicken, 1 tsp canola mayo, and tangerine and avocado slices (406 calories)	4 oz Seared Wild Salmon with 1 Tbsp Summer Pesto (recipe p. 286) 1 cup Grated Celery Root Salad (recipe p. 275) ½ cup Pan-Seared Brussels Sprouts with Gruyère (recipe p. 281) (561 calories)
WEDNESDAY	½ cup Warm Pumpkin Oatmeal (recipe p. 273) topped with 2 Tbsp dried local cherries (or other dried local fruit) and 2 Tbsp walnuts, and drizzled with 1 tsp maple syrup (386 calories)	Winter Endive Salad with 2 oz extra Roasted Rosemary Chicken (recipe p. 280), ½ cup beans, 1 Tbsp cashews, 1 Tbsp sunflower seeds, 2 Tbsp dried cherries, 2 Tbsp red onion, and ⅓ cup tangerine with 1 Tbsp extra Pomegranate Vinaigrette (449 calories)	½ Frittata with ⅔ cup Roasted Fall Vegetables (recipe p. 275) 1½ cups Chopped Watercress Salad with 1 Tbsp pistachios and 2 tsp extra Pomegranate Vinaigrette 1 slice crusty local bread (395 calories)

	BREAKFAST	LUNCH	DINNER
THURSDAY	1½ cups Gorgeous Green Smoothie (recipe p. 273) 1 oz raw almonds (319 calories)	1½ cups extra Hearty Winter Bean Chili 1 slice toasted extra Pumpkin Cranberry Loaf (446 calories)	1 cup Whole Wheat Penne with Roasted Cauliflower and 1 Tbsp Kale Almond Pesto (recipe p. 284) 2 cups Endive and Avocado Salad with 1 Tbsp Lemon Dressing (recipe p. 279) (682 calories)
FRIDAY	1 slice toasted extra Pumpkin Cranberry Loaf 1 cup nonfat Greek yogurt with 2 Tbsp chopped almonds ½ grapefruit (466 calories)	⅔ cup Eggless Egg Salad sandwich in small whole wheat pita (recipe p. 280) 1 cup chopped watercress with Orange and Avocado Slices (recipe p. 279) 2 tsp extra Pomegranate Vinaigrette (388 calories)	4 oz Steamed Fish with 1 Tbsp extra Kale Almond Pesto (recipe p. 285) ⅔ cup Warm Pink Lentils (recipe p. 283) ½ cup extra Pan-Seared Brussels Sprouts with Gruyère (554 calories)
SATURDAY	1 multigrain waffle ¼ cup extra Cinnamon Apple Compote 1 tsp warm maple syrup 1 soy sausage (238 calories)	1 cup extra Whole Wheat Penne with Roasted Cauliflower and 1 Tbsp Kale Almond Pesto 1 tangerine (500 calories)	1⅔ cups Butternut Squash Pear Bisque (recipe p. 276) 1 slice toasted local bread 1½ cups extra Grated Celery Root Salad (515 calories)
SUNDAY	⅔ cup of your favorite whole grain cereal with ½ cup soymilk, 2 Tbsp almonds, 1 chopped tangerine, and 1 Tbsp sunflower seeds (302 calories)	1⅓ cups extra Butternut Squash Pear Bisque 8 whole grain crackers 2 cups Endive and Avocado Salad with 1 Tbsp Lemon Dressing (559 calories)	4 oz Pork Tenderloin with 2 Tbsp extra Pomegranate Vinaigrette (recipe p. 283) ⅔ cup extra Warm Pink Lentils ½ cup Pureed Sweet Potatoes with Lime (recipe p. 282) (465 calories)

Spring Recipes

WARM BARLEY AND QUINOA PORRIDGE WITH SOYMILK

The beauty of this easy recipe is that you can make it in a slow cooker overnight. Or if you have time, make it in the morning. Quinoa provides high-quality protein and iron, and the barley's low glycemic index helps give it staying power all morning.

½ cup barley

½ cup quinoa

1 cinnamon stick

4 cups water

Pinch of salt

2½ cups soymilk

5 tablespoons chopped walnuts

2½ cups fresh cherries

5 teaspoons raw local honey or maple syrup

1. Place the barley, quinoa, cinnamon stick, water, and salt in a slow cooker and cook on low overnight. Alternately, combine them in a medium saucepan, bring to a boil, then cover, lower the heat, and simmer until tender, about 40 minutes.

2. Serve each portion topped with ½ cup soymilk, 1 tablespoon walnuts, ½ cup cherries, and 1 teaspoon honey.

MAKES 5 SERVINGS (1 CUP EACH)

Per serving: 307 calories, 10 g protein, 49 g carbohydrates, 9 g fat, 0 mg cholesterol, 6 g fiber, 64 mg sodium

MULTIGRAIN PANCAKES

Enjoy 2 small to medium pancakes from your favorite whole grain pancake mix that has a clean ingredient list. Prepare in a nonstick pan with 1 teaspoon canola oil.

POACHED EGG WITH SPINACH

If you're not a huge spinach fan, enjoy this dish with ½ cup cooked asparagus instead.

1 teaspoon olive oil

2 cups fresh spinach

1 clove garlic, minced

Pinch of salt and freshly cracked pepper

½ whole wheat English muffin

1 egg, poached

1. Warm the oil in a medium saucepan. Add the spinach and garlic and cook, stirring frequently, until wilted. Season with the salt and pepper.

2. Place the spinach mixture on top of the English muffin and top with the poached egg. Shower with pepper and serve.

MAKES 1 SERVING

Per serving: 200 calories, 11 g protein, 20 g carbohydrates, 10 g fat, 225 mg cholesterol, 4 g fiber, 283 mg sodium

---

SOUTHWEST TOFU SCRAMBLE

1 teaspoon olive oil

1 scallion, chopped

⅔ cup soft tofu

Pinch of garlic powder or dried chili powder (optional)

⅓ cup black beans, rinsed and drained

2 tablespoons jarred local or regional salsa

Warm the oil in a small saucepan over medium-high heat. Add the scallion and cook for about 2 minutes. Add the tofu and "scramble" (just like you would an egg) until heated through, about 2 minutes. Add garlic powder to taste, if desired. Enjoy with the black beans and salsa.

MAKES 1 SERVING

Per serving: 247 calories, 16 g protein, 1 g carbohydrates, 11 g fat, 0 mg cholesterol, 7 g fiber, 390 mg sodium

MINTY SPINACH PEA SOUP

Both the vibrant green color and the bright flavor shout spring. This soup also works well using frozen veggies if it's still too early in the season. I've even used frozen pearl onions in a moment of desperation, and it was fantastic!

1 tablespoon olive oil

1 large spring onion, chopped (about ½ cup)

1 bunch scallions, chopped

2 cups fresh or frozen peas

5 cups chicken or vegetable broth (bouillon or concentrate, if possible)

1 large bunch spinach, stems removed, or about 10 ounces fresh baby spinach

½ cup plain low-fat organic yogurt

Salt and freshly cracked pepper

½ bunch mint leaves, chopped

1. Warm the oil in a large saucepan over medium heat. Add the spring onion and scallions and cook, stirring frequently, for 5 to 6 minutes, or until soft.

2. Add the peas and broth and bring to a boil. Reduce the heat and simmer for about 10 minutes. Add the spinach and stir. Heat until cooked through, about 3 to 4 minutes.

3. Puree the soup in batches in a blender or food processor (or use an immersion blender).

4. Add the yogurt, taste, and adjust seasonings with salt and pepper. Swirl in the mint and serve.

MAKES 6 SERVINGS (1½ CUPS EACH)

Per serving: 125 calories, 6 g protein, 19 g carbohydrates, 3 g fat, 2 mg cholesterol, 7 g fiber, 479 mg sodium

SPRING LETTUCE SALAD WITH TUSCAN LEMON VINAIGRETTE

Enjoy unlimited local spring greens tossed with 1 tablespoon of Tuscan Lemon Vinaigrette (below).

MAKES 1 SERVING

Per serving: 108 calories, 1 g protein, 3 g carbohydrates, 11 g fat, 0 mg cholesterol, 2 g fiber, 14 mg sodium

---

TUSCAN LEMON VINAIGRETTE

There are lots of basic versions of this recipe, but I like adding the garlic for flavor and health.

½ cup extra virgin olive oil

2 tablespoons fresh lemon juice

1 teaspoon grainy mustard

1 small clove garlic, minced

Salt and freshly cracked pepper

Whisk together the olive oil, lemon juice, mustard, and garlic. Season to taste with salt and pepper. Refrigerate in an airtight container for up to 2 weeks.

MAKES ⅔ CUP, 11 SERVINGS (1 TABLESPOON EACH)

Per serving: 88 calories, 0 g protein, 0.5 g carbohydrates, 10 g fat, 0 mg cholesterol, 0 g fiber, 50 mg sodium

SESAME GINGER VINAIGRETTE

This recipe is courtesy of Chef Keith Snow from Harvest Eating. It lights up in your mouth and is incredibly versatile. Try it on salads, veggies, fish, and poultry. For a milder flavor, use canola oil in place of olive oil.

3 tablespoons sesame oil

¾ cup olive oil

1 whole clove garlic

3 tablespoons seasoned rice wine vinegar

2 tablespoons lime juice

2 tablespoons minced fresh ginger

4 tablespoons chopped cilantro

2 tablespoons toasted sesame oil

3 tablespoons minced shallot

Grated zest of 1 lime

Pinch of salt and freshly cracked black pepper

Place all ingredients in a blender and whirl to emulsify the dressing.

MAKES ABOUT 1¾ CUPS, 28 SERVINGS (1 TABLESPOON EACH)

Per serving: 77 calories, 0 g protein, 1 g carbohydrates, 9 g fat, 0 mg cholesterol, 0 g fiber, 38 mg sodium

---

ASPARAGUS SALAD WITH SESAME GINGER VINAIGRETTE

This recipe is courtesy of Chef Keith Snow from Harvest Eating.

1 bunch asparagus, steamed until just cooked (place in a bath of cold water to stop the cooking and retain its vibrant green color), cooled and cut into 1" lengths

3 tablespoons Sesame Ginger Vinaigrette (above)

3 cups washed and spun dry local lettuce (preferably organic)

¼ cup finely diced carrot

Salt and pepper

1. Toss the asparagus in 1 tablespoon of the vinaigrette to coat.

2. Add the lettuce, carrot, the remaining 2 tablespoons of vinaigrette, and salt and pepper to taste. Toss gently. Taste and adjust the seasoning as needed.

MAKES 2 SERVINGS

Per serving: 151 calories, 4 g protein, 0 g carbohydrates, 12 g fat, 0 mg cholesterol, 5 g fiber, 67 mg sodium

GARLICKY EDAMAME HUMMUS

Garnish this bright green, good-for-you dip with a drizzle of olive oil, a splash of fresh lemon juice, or a pinch of paprika for added wow.

1½ cups edamame (cooked according to package directions)

juice of 1 lemon

zest of 1 lemon

¼ cup water

2 tablespoons tahini

2 cloves garlic, smashed

½ teaspoon salt

1 teaspoon cumin

¼ teaspoon coriander

¼ cup chopped fresh parsley

2 tablespoons olive oil

1. Combine edamame, lemon juice, lemon zest, water, tahini, garlic, salt, cumin, coriander, and parsley in a food processor and puree until smooth. With the motor running, add the olive oil and continue pureeing until the oil is incorporated and the hummus is smooth. Taste and adjust seasonings as necessary. Thin with a bit of water if necessary.

2. Serve on toasted pita crisps or with all-natural whole-grain crackers.

MAKES 15 SERVINGS (2 TABLESPOONS)

Per serving: 50 calories, 2.5 g protein, 3 g carbohydrates, 3.5 g fat, 0 mg cholesterol, 0.5 g fiber, 94 mg sodium

---

GRILLED ASPARAGUS WITH LEMON

Enjoy 1 bunch of asparagus grilled with 2 teaspoons olive oil, and unlimited lemon juice and a pinch of salt and pepper.

MAKES 1–2 SERVINGS (1 CUP EACH)

Per serving: 105 calories, 4 g protein, 24 g carbohydrates, 7 g fat, 0 mg cholesterol, 4 g fiber, 50 mg sodium

SWEET TARRAGON DRESSING

Our family friend, Jennifer Weston, a personal chef extraordinaire from Jackson Hole, Wyoming, shared this recipe with me. Use it to shed carbon and the hopelessly long ingredient lists of store-bought versions of salad dressing.

> 1½ teaspoons salt
>
> ¾ teaspoon hot-pepper sauce
>
> ¼ cup sugar
>
> ¼ cup tarragon vinegar
>
> ¾ cup canola oil

In a small bowl, whisk together all of the ingredients. Refrigerate in an airtight container for up to 2 weeks.

MAKES 1½ CUPS, 24 SERVINGS (1 TABLESPOON EACH)

Per serving: 70 calories, 0 g protein, 2 g carbohydrates, 7 g fat, 0 mg cholesterol, 0 g fiber, 50 mg sodium

---

SPINACH SALAD WITH STRAWBERRIES, ALMONDS, AND POPPY SEEDS

Strawberries arrive in late spring in many parts of the United States, so I've included one strawberry recipe as a nod to this delicious addition to the season.

> 2 cups fresh baby spinach
>
> 1 cup sliced organic local strawberries
>
> 2 tablespoons chopped almonds, toasted lightly
>
> 1 teaspoon poppy seeds
>
> 1 tablespoon Sweet Tarragon Dressing (above)

Combine all ingredients in a bowl and mix well.

MAKES 2 SERVINGS

Per serving: 133 calories, 3 g protein, 14 g carbohydrates, 8 g fat, 0 mg cholesterol, 5 g fiber, 277 mg sodium

BABY BEETS WITH ORANGE ZEST

> 1 cup steamed baby beets (you can keep the skins on when they're this small, which saves time and adds even more taste)
>
> 1 teaspoon grated orange zest
>
> 1 tablespoon fresh orange juice
>
> Pinch of salt and freshly cracked pepper

Combine all ingredients in a small bowl and mix. Taste and adjust seasoning if necessary.

MAKES 1 SERVING

Per serving: 106 calories, 4 g protein, 24 g carbohydrates, less than 1 g fat, 0 mg cholesterol, 9 g fiber, 300 mg sodium

---

HUMMUS WRAP

Enjoy ½ cup hummus in a small whole wheat wrap with 1 cup chopped or shredded spring vegetables.

MAKES 1 SERVING

Per serving: 376 calories, 17 g protein, 46 g carbohydrates, 15 g fat, 0 mg cholesterol, 12 g fiber, 646 mg sodium

---

GRILLED VEGGIE BURGER IN WHOLE WHEAT PITA POCKET

Enjoy your favorite grilled veggie burger in a whole wheat pita with your favorite grainy mustard. Tuck in 1 cup baby spring greens, or ½ cup of your favorite seasonal chopped or shredded veggies.

MAKES 1 SERVING

Per serving: 311 calories, 18 g protein, 49 g carbohydrates, 6 g fat, 1 mg cholesterol, 10 g fiber, 659 mg sodium

SPRING ORZO PASTA WITH EDAMAME

In Italy, you know it's spring when fava beans hit the markets. However, since they're a bit hard to come by in some places here, I've used edamame in this dish instead to boost the protein, fiber, and phytonutrient content. If you are lucky enough to live in a place with spring mushrooms, by all means cook them along with the onions.

1 pound orzo pasta

1 cup edamame

1 cup fresh or frozen peas

2 tablespoons olive oil

1 yellow or white spring onion, or 1 bunch scallions, sliced

1 cup steamed asparagus spears, cut into 1" pieces

3 tablespoons chopped fresh lemon thyme (or regular) or parsley

Grated zest of 1 lemon

¼ cup pine nuts, toasted

Salt and freshly cracked pepper

2 tablespoons freshly grated Parmesan cheese

1. In a medium pot of lightly salted water, cook the orzo according to the package directions. During the final 4 to 5 minutes, add the edamame and peas and cook. Drain, but reserve ½ cup of the cooking liquid.

2. Meanwhile, warm the oil in a medium saucepan over medium-high heat. Add the onion and cook for 5 to 8 minutes, or until soft. Remove from the heat.

3. In a separate saucepan, steam the asparagus until crisp tender, about 4 to 5 minutes (if you want to retain their bright color, shock them in a bowl of cold water).

4. Add the drained orzo mixture to the saucepan with the onions. Add the thyme, lemon zest, and pine nuts and combine. Season with salt and pepper. Add the reserved cooking liquid, if necessary, to loosen the pasta.

5. Ladle into bowls and top with the Parmesan.

MAKES 5 SERVINGS

Per serving: 538 calories, 21 g protein, 79 g carbohydrates, 16 g fat, 4 mg cholesterol, 9 g fiber, 66 mg sodium

TOFU CASHEW STIR-FRY WITH SUGAR SNAP PEAS

I like to add cashews to a stir-fry because they add texture, crunch, heart-healthy fats, and a bit more staying power. If you have any extra asparagus on hand, that goes nicely in here, too. Serve with 1 cup steamed brown rice topped with 2 tablespoons chopped scallions.

1 block (16 ounces) extra-firm tofu, cut into squares

½ cup low-sodium marinade of your choice, or ¼ cup Sesame Ginger Vinaigrette (page 240)

1 tablespoon canola oil

½ teaspoon toasted sesame oil

Pinch of red-pepper flakes (optional)

2 to 3 scallions, chopped

1 clove garlic, minced

1 pound sugar snap peas, strung

1 tablespoon water

¼ cup raw cashews, lightly toasted

¼ cup chopped cilantro

1. Marinate the tofu in marinade of your choice for several hours or overnight.

2. In a wok or a large skillet, heat the canola oil, sesame oil, and red-pepper flakes, if desired, over medium-high heat. Add the scallions and garlic and cook for 2 minutes. Add the snap peas and water. Continue to cook, stirring frequently, for about 3 minutes.

3. Add the tofu and the marinade and cook until heated through, 2 to 3 minutes. Remove from the heat. Top with the cashews and cilantro.

MAKES 4 SERVINGS

Per serving: 284 calories, 17 g protein, 19 g carbohydrates, 17 g fat, 0 mg cholesterol, 7 g fiber, 11 mg sodium

SPICY TOFU TACOS

These can absolutely be made as "not so spicy tofu tacos" if that's how you prefer them—just tone down the amount of pepper and chili powder you use. Use this recipe in summer, too, but loaded with chopped local tomatoes and other fixings from your farmers' market.

1 tablespoon canola oil

1 package (16 ounces) extra-firm tofu, crumbled

2 cloves garlic, minced

½ cup chopped onion

2 teaspoons chili powder

½ teaspoon paprika

¼ teaspoon ground red pepper

1 teaspoon ground cumin

¼ teaspoon salt

1 to 2 teaspoons fresh lime juice

½ cup stewed tomatoes

1 cup steamed brown rice

¼ cup chopped cilantro

8 all-natural whole wheat soft taco shells, warmed

2 cups chopped local lettuce

1 bunch scallions, chopped

½ cup jarred local or regional salsa

½ cup chopped ripe olives

¼ cup local sharp cheese, shredded

1. Warm the oil in a large saucepan over medium heat. Add the tofu, garlic, and onion and cook until the onions are soft, about 5 to 6 minutes. Add the chili powder, paprika, red pepper, cumin, salt, lime juice, and tomatoes to the skillet and stir. Cook for 3 minutes. Stir in the rice and cilantro.

2. Spoon ½ cup of the tofu mixture into each taco shell. Top each taco with unlimited lettuce and scallions, 1 tablespoon salsa, 1 tablespoon olives, and 1½ teaspoons cheese.

MAKES 4 SERVINGS (2 TACOS EACH)

Per serving: 516 calories, 21 g protein, 60 g carbohydrates, 20 g fat, 6 mg cholesterol, 8 g fiber, 984 mg sodium

GRILLED CAJUN SHRIMP SKEWERS

Choose your favorite low-sodium Cajun spice rub, preferred herbs, or seafood rub and sprinkle on US-farmed shrimp. Enjoy with Baby Beets with Orange Zest (page 243) on unlimited spring lettuce, and 1 cup extra Spring Orzo Pasta with Edamame (page 244).

MAKES 1 SERVING

Per serving (shrimp only): 514 calories, 43 g protein, 64 g carbohydrates, 11 g fat, 232 mg cholesterol, 13 g fiber, 825 mg sodium

---

GINGER CHICKEN KEBABS

½ cup honey

2 tablespoons minced garlic

¼ cup peeled and grated fresh ginger

4 tablespoons soy sauce

2 organic local boneless, skinless chicken breasts, cut into 1½" cubes (about 1 pound)

1. In a small saucepan, combine the honey, garlic, ginger, and soy sauce and warm over low heat until the honey is just melted.

2. Place the chicken in a shallow pan and pour the soy-honey mixture over it. Mix well. Cover and refrigerate overnight.

3. Soak bamboo skewers, if using, in water for 30 minutes so they don't burn.

4. Prepare the grill. Thread the chicken pieces onto skewers and cook, covered, over medium-high heat until cooked through.

MAKES 4 SERVINGS

Per serving: 204 calories, 17 g protein, 28 g carbohydrates, 2 g fat, 38 mg cholesterol, 2 g fiber, 811 mg sodium

WILD GAME BURGERS

1 pound ground venison, elk, or grass-fed bison

½ cup bread crumbs

1 teaspoon granulated garlic

2 tablespoons all-natural ketchup

½ cup finely chopped (or grated) onion

1 teaspoon dried basil or 1 tablespoon fresh chopped herbs of choice

½ teaspoon salt

Freshly ground pepper

4 medium whole wheat buns (or local whole grain rolls also work well)

Mustard or ketchup

Sliced local onion

Lettuce

1. Heat the grill. Combine the meat, bread crumbs, garlic, ketchup, onion, basil, salt, and pepper and mix well. Shape into 4 small patties. Grill until medium rare (or medium at the most; you don't want them to dry out).

2. Place each burger on a bun and season with 2 teaspoons mustard or ketchup, onion, and lettuce.

MAKES 4 BURGERS

Per burger: 440 calories, 27 g protein, 35 g carbohydrates, 21 g fat, 79 mg cholesterol, 5 g fiber, 772 mg sodium

---

APRICOT STUFFED WITH GOAT CHEESE

1 teaspoon fresh local goat cheese

1 apricot, sliced in half, pit removed

1 teaspoon raw local honey

Place ½ teaspoon of the goat cheese in each half of the apricot. Drizzle with the honey.

MAKES 1 SERVING

Per serving: 58 calories, 1 g protein, 9 g carbohydrates, 1 g fat, 3 mg cholesterol, 0 g fiber, 21 mg sodium

RHUBARB COMPOTE

A versatile hallmark of spring eating that most people associate only with pie, rhubarb has a scant 26 calories per cup yet supplies nearly 10 percent of your daily fiber requirement, as well as vitamin C and calcium.

3 stalks fresh rhubarb, washed and chopped into ½" pieces

½ cup fresh orange juice

¼ cup maple syrup

1 teaspoon cinnamon

1 teaspoon grated fresh ginger (optional)

In a medium saucepan, combine the rhubarb, orange juice, maple syrup, cinnamon, and ginger, if desired, and bring to a boil. Cover, reduce the heat to low, and simmer, stirring occasionally, until the rhubarb is soft, about 5 minutes. Add more maple syrup for sweetness if needed. Can be stored for several days in the fridge, and served warm or at room temperature.

MAKES 3 SERVINGS (½ CUP EACH)

Per serving: 98 calories, 1 g protein, 24 g carbohydrates, 0 g fat, 0 mg cholesterol, 2 g fiber, 44 mg sodium

Summer Recipes

SUMMER SMOOTHIE

Follow the basic Gorgeous Green Smoothie recipe (page 273), but use 1 cup of your favorite local fresh berries instead of frozen, or ½ cup chopped local peach with ½ cup berries.

MAKES 2 SERVINGS

Per serving: 154 calories, 7 g protein, 25 g carbohydrates, 3 g fat, 0 mg cholesterol, 4 g fiber, 96 mg sodium

CHILLED OATMEAL WITH SUMMER FRUIT

Enjoy 1 cup chilled prepared oatmeal topped with ¼ cup soymilk, 1 tablespoon chopped almonds, 1 tablespoon sunflower seeds, and ½ cup fresh local berries or other fruit.

MAKES 1 SERVING

Per serving: 351 calories, 12 g protein, 53 g carbohydrates, 12 g fat, 0 mg cholesterol, 11 g fiber, 198 mg sodium

FALAFEL IN PITA

Tuck 2 pieces of falafel (prepared from a mix such as Fantastic) into a whole wheat pita pocket. Add unlimited chopped local cucumbers, tomatoes, and lettuce. Drizzle with 2 tablespoons nonfat Greek yogurt. Add some cumin or paprika for additional spice, if desired.

MAKES 1 SERVING

Per serving: 310 calories, 13 g protein, 51 g carbohydrates, 8 g fat, 1 mg cholesterol, 7 g fiber, 466 mg sodium

HERBED ZUCCHINI FRITTATA

Enjoy a wedge of this with 1½ cups steamed green beans tossed with a large smashed clove of garlic, ½ teaspoon olive oil, and a pinch of sea salt. By mixing the warm beans with the garlic, you'll infuse them with flavor quickly.

> **1 tablespoon olive oil**
>
> **½ small onion, diced**
>
> **1 clove garlic, chopped**
>
> **1 large (or 2 small) local zucchini, cut into quarters lengthwise and sliced**
>
> **Salt and freshly cracked pepper**
>
> **6 organic local eggs, beaten**
>
> **2 heaping tablespoons chopped mixed herbs (such as chives, basil, parsley, and lemon thyme)**

1. Preheat the oven to 500°F.

2. In a medium ovenproof skillet (such as a cast-iron skillet), warm the olive oil over medium heat. Make sure the oil coats the entire pan to prevent sticking (alternately, use a tiny spritz of a canola or olive oil spray).

3. Add the onion and cook, stirring frequently, for 3 to 5 minutes, or until soft.

4. Add the garlic and zucchini and cook for 5 to 8 minutes, stirring occasionally, until cooked through and slightly browned on the edges. Add a pinch of salt and pepper to taste.

5. Spread out the zucchini mixture evenly on the bottom of the pan. Gently pour in the eggs and sprinkle with the herbs. Continue to cook over medium heat until the frittata is set on the sides, about 3 to 4 minutes.

6. Transfer the frittata to the oven to "finish" off the top, about 1 to 2 minutes. The frittata is ready when it looks completely cooked (as opposed to runny) and is puffed slightly.

7. Remove with a pot holder and set aside to cool for about 5 minutes. You can slice and serve as you would a pie.

MAKES 2 SERVINGS

Per serving: 288 calories, 22 g protein, 7 g carbohydrates, 22 g fat, 675 mg cholesterol, 1 g fiber, 257 mg sodium

EASY GAZPACHO

If chopping vegetables sounds like too much work, place larger cut pieces into a food processor (do each veggie separately) and "pulse" until they're more coarsely chopped; transfer to a bowl before processing the next vegetable. Just be sure not to pulverize them.

1 cucumber, diced

1 local red bell pepper, diced

½ cup finely chopped red onion

4 ripe tomatoes (about 1½ pounds), chopped

3 cups low-sodium tomato juice

2 cloves garlic, minced

2 tablespoons olive oil

2–4 tablespoons balsamic vinegar or lemon juice

Salt and freshly cracked pepper

2 tablespoons chopped parsley or cilantro (optional)

Place the cucumber, bell pepper, onion, tomatoes, tomato juice, garlic, and olive oil in a large bowl and mix well. Add 2 tablespoons of the vinegar and the salt and pepper to taste. Add a bit more vinegar if you need to brighten the flavors further. Cover and refrigerate for at least 2 hours before serving. Then ladle into bowls and garnish with the parsley, if desired.

MAKES 5 SERVINGS (1⅓ CUPS EACH)

Per serving: 131 calories, 3 g protein, 18 g carbohydrates, 6 g fat, 0 mg cholesterol, 3 g fiber, 90 mg sodium

TABBOULEH SALAD WITH WHITE BEANS

What's not to love about tabbouleh? There's no cooking involved, and it's super versatile either in salads, along grilled local organic meat and poultry, or tucked into pitas. Though tabbouleh is already a fantastic source of fiber, I've added white beans to boost the protein. Garbanzo beans work great here, too.

1 cup bulgur wheat

1½ cups boiling water

¼ cup fresh lemon juice

1 teaspoon lemon zest

½ cup olive oil

1½ teaspoons salt

Freshly cracked pepper

1 cup finely chopped scallion (or ½ cup chopped local red onion)

1 cucumber, diced

2–3 tomatoes, seeded and chopped (about 2 cups)

1 can (15 ounces) white beans, rinsed and drained

⅔ cup chopped mint

1 bunch parsley, chopped (about 1 cup)

1. Place the bulgur in a large mixing bowl. Pour the boiling water over it. Add the lemon juice and zest, olive oil, salt, and pepper and mix well. Allow to sit for about an hour, until the bulgur is tender and fluffy.

2. Add the scallion, cucumber, tomatoes, beans, and parsley and mix well. Taste and adjust the seasoning if necessary; a bit more lemon juice will brighten the flavors even more.

MAKES 8–10 SERVINGS (1 CUP EACH)

Per serving: 242 calories, 7 g protein, 28 g carbohydrates, 13 g fat, 0 mg cholesterol, 8 g fiber, 401 mg sodium

FARM SALAD WITH HARD-BOILED EGG

Enjoy unlimited summer lettuce greens with 1 cup chopped vegetables from your CSA or farmers' market. Add 1 sliced hard-boiled local egg and drizzle with 2 tablespoons Tuscan Lemon Vinaigrette (page 239) or Sweet Tarragon Dressing (page 242).

MAKES 1 SERVING

Per serving: 317 calories, 14 g protein, 12 g carbohydrates, 27 g fat, 225 mg cholesterol, 6 g fiber, 112 mg sodium

---

FARM SALAD WITH BEANS AND FINGERLING POTATOES

Enjoy unlimited summer lettuce greens with 1 cup chopped vegetables from your CSA or farmers' market. Add ½ cup beans (kidney, chickpea, or navy) and ⅓ cup sliced fingerling potatoes, and drizzle with 2 tablespoons Tuscan Lemon Vinaigrette (page 239).

MAKES 1 SERVING

Per serving: 441 calories, 19 g protein, 48 g carbohydrates, 23 g fat, 0 mg cholesterol, 17 g fiber, 667 mg sodium

---

CUMIN LIME HUMMUS

1 can (15 ounces) chickpeas, rinsed and drained

1 clove garlic, minced

2 teaspoons fresh lime juice

1 teaspoon ground cumin

½ teaspoon salt

3 tablespoons extra virgin olive oil

2 tablespoons water (or tahini, if you have it)

1 tablespoon chopped fresh basil (optional)

1. Place the chickpeas, garlic, lime juice, cumin, and salt in a food processor and process until smooth.

2. With processor running, add the oil, water, and basil (if using), and blend.

3. Taste and adjust seasonings to your liking.

MAKES ABOUT 2¼ CUPS, 18 SERVINGS (2 TABLESPOONS EACH)

Per serving: 50 calories, 1 g protein, 6 g carbohydrates, 3 g fat, 0 mg cholesterol, 1 g fiber, 265 mg sodium

CRUNCHY HERBED PITA TRIANGLES

This is an adaptation of something my mom has made for as long as I can remember—always served with soup in the summertime. It's totally delicious, and you can experiment with the herbs and even spices that you add.

1 whole wheat pita, cut into triangles and then pulled open completely into each "half" (so you have a bunch of single-layer triangles)

1 tablespoon olive oil

1 ounce freshly grated sharp local cheese or Parmesan cheese

1 tablespoon chopped fresh herbs (such as basil, parsley, and chives)

Preheat the oven to 400°F. Lay the pita triangles on a baking sheet and brush each one with a bit of the olive oil. Sprinkle with the cheese and herbs. Bake until just crisp, about 5 minutes.

MAKES 2 SERVINGS

Per serving: 207 calories, 7 g protein, 18 g carbohydrates, 12 g fat, 18 mg cholesterol, 3 g fiber, 356 mg sodium

---

OPEN-FACED TURKEY MELT

1 slice whole grain local bread

3 ounces sliced organic local turkey breast

Sliced fresh local tomatoes

Fresh basil, if you have it

1 ounce local sharp cheese, grated or thinly sliced

Freshly cracked black pepper

Preheat the broiler or toaster oven. Lightly toast the bread, then layer the turkey, tomatoes, basil, and cheese on top of it. Return to the broiler or toaster oven and heat until the cheese is melted, about 2 to 3 minutes. Remove and top with pepper. Serve hot.

MAKES 1 SERVING

Per serving: 351 calories, 34 g protein, 17 g carbohydrates, 17 g fat, 88 mg cholesterol, 2 g fiber, 397 mg sodium

STUFFED TOMATOES WITH QUINOA, RAISINS, AND MINT

These taste even better the next day for lunch. You can add ½ cup cooked lentils for more fiber and protein if you have any on hand or a few tablespoons of finely chopped tofu.

4 large ripe but firm tomatoes

1 teaspoon olive oil, plus additional for drizzling

½ local onion, finely chopped (about ½ cup)

1 clove garlic, minced

1 cup cooked quinoa or whole wheat couscous

¼ cup chopped fresh parsley

¼ cup chopped fresh mint

⅓ cup currants or raisins

2 tablespoons pine nuts, toasted (almonds are okay too)

Salt and freshly cracked pepper

1. Preheat the oven to 375°F. Gently slice off the top of each tomato and reserve. With a spoon, gently remove the pulp, seeds, and liquid. Chop the pulp and place in a medium bowl.

2. In a small saucepan, warm 1 teaspoon of the olive oil over medium-high heat. Add the onion and garlic and cook, stirring frequently, for about 5 minutes, or until soft. Add to the chopped tomato pulp.

3. Add the quinoa, parsley, mint, raisins, and pine nuts, and season with salt and pepper to taste. Stuff the tomatoes with the filling, replace the tops, drizzle or brush the tops with olive oil, and place in a medium baking dish. Bake for 20 to 30 minutes, until the tomatoes are soft and the filling is hot. Serve warm or at room temperature.

MAKES 4 SERVINGS

Per serving: 164 calories, 6 g protein, 22 g carbohydrates, 7 g fat, 0 mg cholesterol, 5 g fiber, 20 mg sodium

FRESH CORN, PEPPER, AND BLACK BEAN TACOS

Feel free to turn the spices up or down in this recipe. For a quick shortcut, you can also use your favorite low-sodium taco seasoning mix.

2 tablespoons canola oil

½ local onion, chopped

2 cloves garlic, minced

1 cup fresh corn kernels

1 red, yellow, or orange local bell pepper, diced

1 can (15 ounces) black beans, rinsed and drained

2 teaspoons chili powder

½ teaspoon paprika

¼ teaspoon ground red pepper

1 teaspoon ground cumin

¼ teaspoon salt

1–2 teaspoons fresh lime juice

¼ cup chopped cilantro

8 all-natural whole wheat soft taco shells, warmed

2 cups chopped lettuce

½ cup fresh local salsa

1. Warm the oil in a large saucepan over medium heat. Add the onion and garlic and cook, stirring frequently, until the onion is soft, about 5 minutes. Add the corn and bell pepper and cook until tender, about 5 to 6 minutes. Add the beans, chili powder, paprika, ground red pepper, cumin, salt, and lime juice and stir well. Cook for 3 minutes. Taste and adjust the seasonings as needed. Remove from the heat and stir in the cilantro.

2. Spoon ⅔ cup of the bean mixture into the taco shells. Top each taco with ¼ cup lettuce and 1 tablespoon salsa.

MAKES 4 SERVINGS (2 TACOS EACH)

Per serving: 517 calories, 21 g protein, 60 g carbohydrates, 20 g fat, 6 mg cholesterol, 8 g fiber, 984 mg sodium

FRESH PEACH SALSA

4 ripe local peaches, diced

1 jalapeño chile pepper, seeds removed, finely minced (wear plastic gloves when handling)

¼ cup diced red onion

1 tablespoon grated fresh ginger

1 tablespoon lemon or lime juice

Combine all ingredients in a medium bowl and mix well.

MAKES 2 CUPS, 4 SERVINGS (½ CUP EACH)

Per serving: 50 calories, 1 g protein, 12 g carbohydrates, 0 g fat, 0 mg cholesterol, 2 g fiber, 24 mg sodium

---

GRILLED LOCAL PLUMS

Here's a basic recipe you can do with virtually any summer "stone fruit" (plums, peaches, apricots, nectarines, etc.). If you don't have maple syrup available, raw local honey or even real sugar works deliciously as well. You can also experiment with a dash of nutmeg, cinnamon, and cloves if you like.

2 ripe but firm local plums, cut in half and pits removed

1 teaspoon maple syrup (optional)

1. Place the fruit cut side down on a medium-hot grill.

2. Grill until the fruit is heated through and the bottoms are slightly caramelized, about 4 to 5 minutes. Transfer to a plate and drizzle with maple syrup, if desired. Serve warm.

MAKES 1 SERVING

Per serving: 87 calories, 1 g protein, 24 g carbohydrates, 0 g fat, 0 mg cholesterol, 2 g fiber, 1 mg sodium

Fall Recipes

HOT QUINOA CEREAL

This dish provides a protein-rich start to your day. Make a bigger batch and enjoy leftovers the next morning, either chilled (in warmer weather) or reheated.

> 1 medium local pear (preferably organic), diced
>
> Pinch each of clove and nutmeg
>
> ¼ teaspoon cinnamon
>
> ⅔ cup cooked quinoa, prepared with soymilk or organic local milk
>
> 1 tablespoon chopped walnuts

Sprinkle the pear with clove, nutmeg, and cinnamon. Fold into the hot quinoa cereal, top with chopped walnuts, and serve.

MAKES 1 SERVING

Per serving: 349 calories, 10 g protein, 56 g carbohydrates, 12 g fat, 0 mg cholesterol, 12 g fiber, 11 mg sodium

CINNAMON GRANOLA PARFAIT

> ⅓ cup local cinnamon granola or your favorite clean granola
>
> ½ cup nonfat Greek yogurt
>
> 2 tablespoons dried local cherries or other dried fruit
>
> 2 tablespoons sunflower seeds

In a tall glass, layer half of the granola, half of the yogurt, and half of the fruit and seeds. Repeat the layers and serve immediately.

MAKES 1 SERVING

Per serving: 335 calories, 16 g protein, 49 g carbohydrates, 13 g fat, 3 mg cholesterol, 12 g fiber, 81 mg sodium

FRIED LOCAL EGG OPEN-FACED SANDWICH

When tomatoes are still available in early fall, this is a delicious reason to jump out of bed!

> 1 teaspoon olive oil
>
> 1 fresh local egg
>
> 1 thin slice whole grain local bread, toasted
>
> 1 thick slice tomato
>
> Salt and freshly cracked pepper

1. Warm the olive oil in a small skillet over medium heat. Add the egg, cook until set, flip, and cook through.

2. Slide the warm egg on top of the toast, and top with the tomato. Season with salt and pepper to taste.

MAKES 1 SERVING

Per serving: 183 calories, 9 g protein, 18 g carbohydrates, 10 g fat, 225 mg cholesterol, 5 g fiber, 167 mg sodium

---

SHAVED FENNEL SALAD

In winter, this salad is fantastic with a blood orange instead of an apple—and you can use a splash of the fresh blood orange juice in the dressing instead of lemon juice. For best results, make sure the fennel and apple are sliced into similar-size pieces.

> 1 head fennel, cored and thinly sliced
>
> 1 local fresh apple, peeled, cored, and thinly sliced
>
> 2 tablespoons walnuts
>
> 3 teaspoons Tuscan Lemon Vinaigrette (page 239)

Combine all ingredients in a medium bowl. Mix well and serve.

MAKES 2 SERVINGS

Per serving: 177 calories, 3 g protein, 22 g carbohydrates, 10 g fat, 0 mg cholesterol, 7 g fiber, 65 mg sodium

FALL GREEN FRITTATA

This frittata offers a perfect opportunity to use leftover greens. Feel free to add chopped garlic, sautéed onions, or any remaining veggies you have in the fridge. Easy to make, high in protein, and packing in the power of dark leafy greens—what's not to love?

> 1 teaspoon canola or olive oil
>
> 4 eggs, beaten
>
> About ⅔ cup prepared Gorgeous Greens in a Flash (page 265)
>
> 2 tablespoons chopped fresh parsley
>
> Salt and freshly cracked pepper

1. Preheat the broiler.

2. In a medium ovenproof skillet, warm the oil over medium heat and swirl to coat the pan. Add the eggs and cook for 2 minutes.

3. Gently add the greens, spreading them evenly over the eggs. Sprinkle the parsley over the top, and add salt and pepper to taste.

4. Continue to cook until the edges are set and the bottom is cooked, with only about 1 inch of the top part of the egg mixture still soft and liquid, about 2 to 3 minutes.

5. Place the skillet under the broiler for about 1 minute, until browned and puffy. Remove, let cool for about 5 minutes, and serve either hot or at room temperature.

MAKES 2 SERVINGS

Per serving: 208 calories, 16 g protein, 7 g carbohydrates, 15 g fat, 450 mg cholesterol, 3 g fiber, 234 mg sodium

SWEET POTATO PANCAKES

I love the creamy/crunchy contrast of potato pancakes, and this version provides a hefty dose of beta-carotene. And unlike potatoes, which can turn gray while you work, these are more foolproof and provide a slightly sweeter taste. Use these ratios as a guideline for herbed zucchini pancakes in the summertime.

> 1½ pounds sweet potatoes, peeled and grated
>
> 2 eggs, lightly beaten
>
> ½ yellow or white onion, grated or finely diced
>
> 2 tablespoons bread crumbs (from your local whole grain bread) or flour
>
> ½ teaspoon salt
>
> Freshly cracked pepper
>
> 2 tablespoons canola oil

1. In a medium bowl, combine the sweet potatoes with the eggs, onion, bread crumbs, salt, and pepper to taste.

2. In a medium saucepan, warm the oil over medium-high heat. Drop the sweet potato batter by spoonfuls (the pancakes should be about 2 to 3" wide) and cook until browned, about 5 to 6 minutes. Flip and cook an additional 3 to 4 minutes, until lightly browned and cooked through.

3. Drain on paper towels, and repeat with the remaining batter. Serve warm with a local apple compote or applesauce.

MAKES 4 SERVINGS

Per serving: 262 calories, 7 g protein, 38 g carbohydrates, 10 g fat, 113 mg cholesterol, 5 g fiber, 454 mg sodium

AUTUMN SQUASH AND PINTO BEAN CHILI WITH CINNAMON AND CUMIN

This is my modified version of a dish I first fell in love with from Deborah Madison's *Greens* cookbook. Nothing welcomes the tastes of fall better, and the flavors deepen after a day, so leftovers are super tasty.

3 tablespoons canola oil

1 medium onion, diced

2 cloves garlic, chopped

1 teaspoon ground cumin

1 teaspoon oregano

1 teaspoon cinnamon

½ teaspoon ground cloves

1 tablespoon paprika

1 teaspoon salt

3 cups vegetable or chicken broth (using bouillon)

1 can (16 ounces) diced tomatoes (or 1 pound fresh tomatoes, seeded and chopped)

1 large butternut squash, peeled and cut into 1" cubes (about 3 cups)

3 ears fresh corn, kernels cut from stalk (about 1½ cups)

1 can (16 ounces) pinto beans, rinsed and drained

Chopped cilantro or parsley (optional)

1. Heat the oil in a large skillet or Dutch oven over medium-high heat. Add the onion and cook, stirring frequently, until soft, about 4 to 5 minutes.

2. Lower the heat to medium and add the garlic, cumin, oregano, cinnamon, cloves, paprika, and salt. Cook for about 2 minutes, stirring well. (Add a splash of the broth if you need more moisture.)

3. Add the remaining broth, the tomatoes, and the squash. Bring to a simmer and cook for about 25 minutes, until the squash is almost cooked through.

4. Add the corn and the beans and cook for another 5 minutes, until the squash and corn are cooked. Taste and adjust the seasoning as needed.

5. Garnish with the cilantro, if desired, and serve.

MAKES 6–8 SERVINGS (1⅔ CUPS EACH)

Per serving: 219 calories, 7 g protein, 34 g carbohydrates, 7 g fat, 0 mg cholesterol, 8 g fiber, 542 mg sodium

CRUNCHY CURRIED CHICKEN SALAD

Replacing some of the mayo with nonfat yogurt helps trim the overall fat and provides a refreshing tang as well as an extra dose of healthy probiotics to your day.

CHICKEN SALAD

1½ cups cooked chicken, cut into small cubes

1 stalk celery, diced (about ½ cup)

2 tablespoons chopped scallions

½ cup dried cranberries or cherries

½ cup chopped or slivered almonds (if you want deeper flavor, toast them lightly in a pan before adding)

DRESSING

½ cup canola-based mayonnaise

⅔ cup nonfat plain yogurt

½ teaspoon fresh lemon juice

1 teaspoon curry

½ teaspoon salt

¼ teaspoon ground white pepper

1. *To make the chicken salad:* In a medium bowl, combine the chicken, celery, scallions, cranberries, and almonds.

2. *To make the dressing:* In a small bowl, whisk all of the dressing ingredients together.

3. Fold the dressing into the chicken salad and toss gently to combine. Taste and adjust the seasoning as needed. Cover and refrigerate until ready to eat.

MAKES 6 SERVINGS (½ CUP EACH)

Per serving: 283 calories, 14 g protein, 13 g carbohydrates, 20 g fat, 36 mg cholesterol, 2 g fiber, 360 mg sodium

GORGEOUS GREENS IN A FLASH

Loaded with calcium, vitamin K, and lutein, greens are a lean and green superfood. Greens will cook faster if you cut the stems out of them before chopping; just run a knife right along both sides and pull it out.

> 2 tablespoons olive oil
>
> ½ pound kale, rinsed and chopped
>
> ½ pound collard greens, rinsed and chopped
>
> ½ pound Swiss chard, rinsed and chopped
>
> 1 clove garlic, minced
>
> 2 teaspoons balsamic vinegar
>
> Salt and freshly cracked pepper
>
> Handful of chopped walnuts or pine nuts and ¼ cup golden raisins (optional)

1. Heat the oil in a large skillet over medium heat. Add the kale, collard greens, and Swiss chard (it's okay if they are still a bit damp from rinsing).

2. Cook, tossing frequently, until the greens are almost wilted, about 3 minutes. Add the garlic and toss 1 minute more. Add the vinegar and remove from the heat. Toss to mix, and add salt and pepper to taste. If desired, mix in walnuts and raisins.

MAKES 4 SERVINGS

Per serving: 113 calories, 4 g protein, 11 g carbohydrates, 7 g fat, 0 mg cholesterol, 5 g fiber, 150 mg sodium

WARMED BEETS WITH WALNUT OIL AND CHOPPED WALNUTS

There are two easy ways to prepare beets: Place washed beets, whole and unpeeled, in a steamer and steam until tender when pierced with a knife (about 30 to 35 minutes for an average beet, a bit less for smaller ones, a bit more for larger). Alternately, place washed beets, whole and unpeeled, in a medium baking dish, add about ¼" water, and bake at 400°F for about 35 minutes.

Walnut oil is a delicious heart-healthy fat with a nutty flavor. If you have it, a bit of chopped mint, dill, or parsley is a great addition!

1 pound beets (about 4), steamed or baked (see above)

1 tablespoon walnut oil

¼ cup chopped walnuts

½ teaspoon salt

Freshly cracked pepper

Lemon wedges

1. When the beets have cooled, remove the skin (by hand, with a vegetable peeler, or with a kitchen towel; do this over the sink and wash your hands well afterward, as the color runs a bit) and slice into quarters.

2. Place the beet slices in a medium bowl. Drizzle with the walnut oil and add the walnuts, salt, and pepper to taste. Mix well. Serve with lemon wedges (alternately, you can use a splash of red wine vinegar).

MAKES 4 SERVINGS

Per serving: 129 calories, 3 g protein, 12 g carbohydrates, 8 g fat, 0 mg cholesterol, 5 g fiber, 89 mg sodium

WILD RICE STUFFED ACORN SQUASH

The diced tofu adds protein and staying power, while the dried fruit adds a sweet note, and the nutty wild rice is given added crunch with the almonds.

1 large acorn squash

1 tablespoon olive oil

2 teaspoons maple syrup

Salt and freshly cracked pepper

2 cups vegetable or chicken broth

⅔ cup wild rice

½ onion, finely chopped

1 medium stalk celery, chopped

1 clove garlic, minced

1 cup diced extra-firm tofu (drained)

½ cup chopped dried cranberries or cherries

1 tablespoon orange juice

1 tablespoon grated orange zest

⅓ cup chopped parsley

2 tablespoons chopped almonds (I suggest lightly toasting them first; it brings out a deeper flavor)

1. Preheat the oven to 375°F.

2. Cut the acorn squash in half lengthwise, from stem to tip, and scoop out the seeds. Brush the insides with 1 teaspoon each of the olive oil and maple syrup, and season with salt and pepper. Place flat side down in a baking dish. Add about ½" of water to the dish and bake until soft, about 25 minutes.

3. To prepare the wild rice: Bring the broth to a boil, add the rice, stir, and then cover, reduce to a simmer, and cook until fluffy, about 40 minutes.

4. While the rice and squash are cooking, in a small saucepan, cook the onion, celery, and garlic with the remaining 1 teaspoon olive oil for about 5 minutes, until soft. Remove from the heat and add the tofu, cranberries, orange juice and zest, parsley, and almonds. Add the wild rice when it's ready and mix well.

5. Remove the squash from the oven, place on plates, and fill with the wild rice stuffing. Serve hot. Can also be made in advance and covered, chilled, then reheated.

MAKES 2 SERVINGS

Per serving: 468 calories, 14 g protein, 73 g carbohydrates, 16 g fat, 0 mg cholesterol, 10 g fiber, 484 mg sodium

HEARTY CORN MUFFINS

Whole wheat pastry flour is a fantastic trick to use when baking. It adds fiber, vitamins, and antioxidants but still retains a soft and delicious texture.

1 cup unbleached flour

½ cup whole wheat pastry flour

½ cup cornmeal

2 tablespoons sugar

1 teaspoon baking powder

½ teaspoon salt

1 egg, beaten

4 tablespoons canola oil

½ teaspoon vanilla

1 cup 2% milk

1. Preheat the oven to 375°F. Spray a muffin tin with canola spray and set aside.

2. In a mixing bowl, combine the flours, cornmeal, sugar, baking powder, and salt. Stir to combine.

3. In a glass measuring cup or small bowl, combine the egg, canola oil, vanilla, and milk. Mix well.

4. Make a well in the center of the dry ingredients; pour the wet ingredients into the well and stir just to combine (mixture will be slightly lumpy). Fill each cup of the muffin tin ⅔ full.

5. Bake for 20 to 23 minutes, until the muffins are lightly browned and a toothpick inserted into the centers comes out clean.

6. Let the muffins sit for 5 minutes in the pan. Then remove and cool on a wire rack for 10 minutes. Store in an airtight container for up to 5 days.

MAKES 12 MUFFINS

Per muffin: 142 calories, 3 g protein, 20 g carbohydrates, 6 g fat, 20 mg cholesterol, 1 g fiber, 146 mg sodium

ROASTED CARROTS WITH MINT

I love the refreshing contrast of the mint, but other herbs such as parsley, lemon thyme, and dill work equally well here, so use whatever is available. Roasting is a great basic technique that works well with a variety of herb-vegetable combos.

> **8–10 local carrots, washed, peeled, and cut into quarters**
>
> **3 tablespoons olive oil**
>
> **½ teaspoon salt**
>
> **Freshly cracked pepper**
>
> **¼ cup chopped fresh mint and/or parsley leaves**

Preheat the oven to 400°F. Toss the carrots, olive oil, salt, and pepper together on a baking sheet and mix until coated. Roast for 20 to 25 minutes, or until cooked through and slightly browned on the edges. Remove from the oven, pour into a bowl, and toss with the mint and/or parsley.

MAKES 4 SERVINGS

Per serving: 137 calories, 1 g protein, 13 g carbohydrates, 10 g fat, 0 mg cholesterol, 6 g fiber, 356 mg sodium

---

BALSAMIC ONIONS

Enjoy these tasty onions with 4 ounces of your favorite grilled green fish and steamed purple potatoes.

> **2 tablespoons olive oil**
>
> **1 local yellow onion, thinly sliced**
>
> **2 teaspoons balsamic vinegar**
>
> **Salt and freshly ground pepper**

In a medium saucepan, warm the olive oil and cook the onion over medium heat for 10 minutes, stirring occasionally. Add the vinegar and salt and pepper to taste, and continue to cook and stir for about 2 minutes. Taste and adjust the seasoning as necessary.

MAKES 2 SERVINGS (⅓ CUP EACH)

Per serving: 144 calories, <1 g protein, 6 g carbohydrates, 14 g fat, 0 mg cholesterol, 1 g fiber, 4 mg sodium

CHICKPEAS AND TOFU IN INDIAN RED SAUCE

Don't be put off by the long ingredient list; all of the ingredients are easy and quick to add, and together they provide a rich, wonderful flavor. What I love about this delicious recipe, which is from my friend Kristie Henderson, is that you can use it with any kind of protein—tofu, chicken, lamb, chickpeas, even ground turkey.

1 medium onion, quartered

⅓ plus ½ cup water

2 whole cloves

1 whole green cardamom

1 tablespoon canola oil

¼ teaspoon mustard seeds

¼ teaspoon cumin seeds

1 cinnamon stick (about 2" long), broken into pieces

1 whole dried red chile pepper, broken into bits (wear plastic gloves when handling)

1 cup tomato puree or stewed tomatoes

½ cup extra-firm tofu, drained and cubed

½ cup cooked chickpeas, drained and rinsed

Salt

⅛ teaspoon turmeric

2 teaspoons ground coriander

½ teaspoon garam masala

¼ teaspoon chili powder (preferably Indian chili powder)

½ teaspoon dried mango powder (amchoor) (optional)

Chopped onion and cilantro (optional)

1. Place the onion quarters in a blender or food processor with ⅓ cup water. Puree until smooth. Set aside.

2. Gently smash the cloves and cardamom on a cutting board with the side of a chef's knife to release more flavor.

3. Heat the oil in a medium saucepan over medium-high heat.

4. Add the mustard seeds, cumin seeds, cloves, cardamom, cinnamon, and chile pepper, and cook for 1 minute. Then add the pureed onion. Cook, stirring occasionally, for 5 to 7 minutes, or until the onion is soft and the mixture reduces slightly.

5. Add the tomatoes, tofu, chickpeas, remaining ½ cup water, salt to taste, and turmeric and cook for 5 to 7 minutes longer.

6. Add the coriander, garam masala, chili powder, and mango powder, if desired, and cook for 2 minutes longer.

$7.$ Serve hot, garnished with the chopped onion and cilantro, if desired.

MAKES 4 SERVINGS

Per serving: 229 calories, 10 g protein, 30 g carbohydrates, 9 g fat, 0 mg cholesterol, 7 g fiber, 985 mg sodium

---

BUTTERY CABBAGE

In the colder months, I crave heartier flavors. Using a small amount of butter along with the olive oil provides that rich buttery taste but keeps the saturated fat levels in check.

> **1 tablespoon local unsalted butter (preferably organic)**
>
> **1 tablespoon olive oil**
>
> **1 medium head white cabbage, cored and thinly sliced**
>
> **½ teaspoon salt**
>
> **½ teaspoon freshly cracked pepper**

In a large skillet, melt the butter over medium heat. Add the olive oil, cabbage, salt, and pepper, and toss lightly with tongs to combine. Cook until the cabbage is wilted through and slightly browned on the edges, about 10 minutes, stirring occasionally.

MAKES 2–4 SERVINGS (1¼ CUPS EACH)

Per serving: 132 calories, 3 g protein, 15 g carbohydrates, 8 g fat, 9 mg cholesterol, 9 g fiber, 423 mg sodium

WILD VENISON RAGÙ

Venison is so lean that there's typically no need for the step of draining fat from the browned meat. If you don't have access to local wild venison, try using free-range bison meat instead (in which case you may need to drain first). Dried porcini mushrooms add a meaty taste and texture—and are super light to ship—and there are some wonderful sustainable mushroom companies around the country. Mushrooms also have a 365-days-a-year growing season! This dish is truly exceptional spooned over a cup of prepared polenta.

2 tablespoons olive oil

1 onion, chopped

1 carrot, diced

1 stalk celery, diced

2 teaspoons fennel seeds

2 teaspoons oregano

1 pound ground venison or bison

4 cloves garlic, chopped

1 can (28 ounces) stewed tomatoes

2 tablespoons tomato paste

1 bay leaf

3 sprigs thyme

¼ cup red wine

1 teaspoon salt

Freshly cracked pepper

1 ounce dried porcini mushrooms (optional), soaked in hot water for 20 minutes, then diced, or 8 ounces fresh mushrooms

1. In a medium saucepan, warm the olive oil and cook the onion, carrot, celery, fennel seeds, and oregano over medium-high heat until soft, about 5 minutes.

2. Add the venison or bison and the garlic. Lower the heat to medium and continue cooking until the meat is browned. Add the tomatoes, tomato paste, bay leaf, thyme, red wine, salt, pepper to taste, and mushrooms, if desired, and simmer for about 30 to 40 minutes, or until the sauce is reduced and thickened and the flavors have combined. Remove and discard the bay leaf and thyme sprigs.

MAKES 8 SERVINGS

Per serving: 159 calories, 10 g protein, 8 g carbohydrates, 10 g fat, 30 mg cholesterol, 1 g fiber, 424 mg sodium

Winter Recipes

GORGEOUS GREEN SMOOTHIE

Green is just the environmental color of this delicious morning breakfast drink (the blueberries actually make it purple), but it's a nice "green" recipe because it uses soymilk plus local fruit and honey.

1 cup soymilk

2 teaspoons raw local honey (or alternately use ¼ cup deep red juice such as pomegranate, blueberry, cranberry, or cherry juice)

1 teaspoon vanilla extract

¾ cup frozen local blueberries from summer (or frozen naked fruit if store-bought), or if in summer, ¾ cup local fresh fruit (e.g., strawberries and peaches are also delish)

¼ cup nonfat Greek yogurt

½–1 cup crushed ice

MAKES 2 SERVINGS

Per serving: 154 calories, 6 g protein, 26 g carbohydrates, 3 g fat, 1 mg cholesterol, 3 g fiber, 93 mg sodium

WARM PUMPKIN OATMEAL

Prepare ½ cup dry oatmeal with water. When cooked, swirl in 2 tablespoons canned pumpkin and warm through. Top with 2 tablespoons dried local cherries (or other dried local fruit) and 2 tablespoons chopped walnuts. Sweeten with 1 teaspoon maple syrup, if you desire.

MAKES 1 SERVING

Per serving: 386 calories, 11 g protein, 58 g carbohydrates, 13 g fat, 0 mg cholesterol, 10 g fiber, 2 mg sodium

PUMPKIN CRANBERRY LOAF

This recipe is compliments of my friend Melanie Plesko, RD, who is also a trained chef with a passion to seek out flavorful, nutritious, locally grown food. Whole wheat pastry flour is a great staple to have on hand; it has a softer texture than regular whole wheat flour. I usually substitute about half of the white flour called for in recipes with it to boost fiber and nutrients while still keeping baked goods soft and delicious. I often add a handful of chopped walnuts (about ⅓ cup) and ¼ cup dark chocolate chips.

1 cup unbleached flour

1 cup whole wheat pastry flour

2 teaspoons baking powder

½ teaspoon baking soda

1½ teaspoons ground cinnamon

½ teaspoon salt

1 cup sugar

1 cup canned pumpkin

½ cup soymilk

¼ cup unsalted butter, softened (canola oil works well, too)

1 tablespoon grated orange zest

¼ cup fresh orange juice

1 large egg

⅓ cup dried cranberries (or cherries work well, too)

1. Preheat the oven to 350°F. Spray an 8" × 4" loaf pan with canola spray, or lightly brush with canola oil.

2. In a large bowl, combine the flours, baking powder, baking soda, cinnamon, and salt. In another bowl, whisk together the sugar, pumpkin, soymilk, butter, orange zest, orange juice, and egg. Add to the flour mixture and stir just until combined. Then fold in the cranberries.

3. Pour the batter into the prepared loaf pan. Bake for 1 hour, or until a toothpick inserted into the center comes out clean. Let cool for 10 minutes before slicing.

MAKES 1 LOAF (12 SLICES)

Per slice: 201 calories, 3 g protein, 38 g carbohydrates, 5 g fat, 29 mg cholesterol, 3 g fiber, 284 mg sodium

FRITTATA WITH ROASTED FALL VEGETABLES

Follow the directions for the Fall Green Frittata (page 261), but substitute ⅔ cup of the leftover Roasted Fall Vegetables (page 286) instead of the Gorgeous Greens.

MAKES 2 SERVINGS

Per serving: 222 calories, 15 g protein, 11 g carbohydrates, 15 g fat, 450 mg cholesterol, 2 g fiber, 340 mg sodium

---

GRATED CELERY ROOT SALAD

A turniplike root vegetable that has a flavor similar to strong celery combined with parsley, celery root is also known as celeriac. Unlike celery, it must be peeled before preparation. But don't let that discourage you—this salad is fabulous!

> **1 pound celery root, peeled and grated (about 2 cups)**
>
> **4 cups water plus 3 teaspoons lemon juice**
>
> **½ cup Tuscan Lemon Vinaigrette (page 239)**
>
> **½ cup dried local cherries or cranberries**
>
> **½ teaspoon black pepper**

In a large bowl, soak the grated celery root in the water and lemon juice mixture for 15 minutes to prevent browning. Drain. Mix with the vinaigrette, cherries, and pepper. Taste and adjust the seasoning. Chill in the refrigerator for at least 1 hour.

MAKES 7 SERVINGS

Per serving: 159 calories, 1 g protein, 13 g carbohydrates, 12 g fat, 0 mg cholesterol, 2 g fiber, 72 mg sodium

BUTTERNUT SQUASH PEAR BISQUE

Bisque seems so decadent, but the butternut squash provides a rich, creamy texture with very little additional fat. This recipe is from my friend Melanie Plesko, RD, who is also a trained chef with a passion to seek out flavorful, nutritious, locally grown food.

1 butternut squash (about 2 pounds)

1 teaspoon unsalted butter

2 teaspoons olive oil

2 cups chopped peeled Bartlett pears (about 1 pound)

1½ cups thinly sliced yellow onion

2½ cups water

1 cup pear nectar

4 cups vegetable broth

1 tablespoon curry powder

½ teaspoon salt

¼ teaspoon freshly cracked pepper

½ cup local, organic half-and-half

2 tablespoons maple syrup (optional)

2 tablespoons pumpkin seeds, toasted

1. Preheat the oven to 375°F. Cut the squash in half lengthwise and discard the seeds. Place the squash halves, cut side down, on a baking sheet; bake for 45 minutes, or until tender. Cool. Using a spoon, scoop out the flesh into a bowl and mash; set aside.

2. In a Dutch oven, melt the butter over medium-high heat and add the oil. Add the pears and onion and cook, stirring frequently, for 10 minutes, or until lightly browned. Add the reserved squash, the water, nectar, broth, curry powder, salt, and pepper. Bring to a boil, partially cover, reduce the heat, and simmer for 40 minutes. Puree in batches in a blender or food processor. Stir in the half-and-half and maple syrup, if desired.

3. Ladle into bowls, top with the pumpkin seeds, and serve.

MAKES 8 SERVINGS (⅔ CUP EACH)

Per serving: 167 calories, 3 g protein, 33 g carbohydrates, 4 g fat, 7 mg cholesterol, 6 g fiber, 392 mg sodium

HEARTY WINTER BEAN CHILI

This recipe is super easy, and it makes tasty leftovers. And it's another great "bridge dish" to help meat-eaters feel satisfied; you can omit 1 can of beans and add ½ pound ground wild game, or even add a package of "meat crumbles" from your freezer section for the appearance and texture of meat. Since the peppers are out of season (hence, higher carbon), you could make an even greener version by substituting butternut squash instead.

3 tablespoons olive oil

1 large onion, diced

3 cloves garlic, minced

1 red bell pepper, chopped

1 green bell pepper, chopped

1 teaspoon ground cumin

1 teaspoon oregano

1 tablespoon chili powder

1 tablespoon paprika

½ teaspoon salt

Freshly cracked black pepper

Pinch of ground red pepper

1 can (15 ounces) pinto beans, rinsed and drained

1 can (15 ounces) black beans, rinsed and drained

1 can (28 ounces) stewed tomatoes

Chopped cilantro or onions (optional)

1. In a large saucepan or Dutch oven, warm the olive oil over medium heat and cook the onion, stirring frequently, for 5 minutes.

2. Add the garlic, bell peppers, cumin, oregano, chili powder, paprika, salt, black pepper to taste, and ground red pepper, and continue to cook until softened, about 4 to 5 minutes.

3. Add the beans and tomatoes and bring to a simmer. Simmer gently for about 20 minutes, or until the flavors have combined. Taste and adjust the seasonings, and serve garnished with cilantro or onions, if desired.

MAKES 6 SERVINGS (1½ CUPS EACH)

Per serving: 245 calories, 9 g protein, 34 g carbohydrates, 8 g fat, 0 mg cholesterol, 9 g fiber, 942 mg sodium

CHOPPED WATERCRESS SALAD

Enjoy 1½ cups of chopped watercress drizzled with 2 teaspoons Pomegranate Vinaigrette (below) and 1 tablespoon pistachios.

MAKES 1 SERVING

Per serving: 63 calories, 3 g protein, 4 g carbohydrates, 5 g fat, 0 mg cholesterol, 1 g fiber, 29 mg sodium

---

POMEGRANATE VINAIGRETTE

This recipe comes compliments of my friend chef Keith Snow from Harvest Eating. He specifically suggests using bulk olive oil in this recipe, as the flavor of extra virgin is a bit too strong for the dressing (you could use canola oil instead). He's an absolute whiz at making seasonal eating tasty, easy, and fun.

¾ cup pomegranate juice

1 tablespoon Dijon mustard

1 small shallot, minced

1 clove garlic, minced

1 tablespoon lemon juice

Pinch of kosher salt

Freshly cracked black pepper

¼ cup olive oil

1. Simmer the pomegranate juice in a small saucepan until reduced to ¼ cup. Cool.

2. Add the mustard, shallot, garlic, and lemon juice. Whisk well.

3. Season with salt and pepper to taste. Slowly drizzle the olive oil into the vinaigrette, whisking constantly, until emulsified. Can be stored, covered tightly, in the fridge for up to a week.

MAKES ABOUT ½ CUP, 12 SERVINGS (2 TEASPOONS EACH)

Per serving: 19 calories, 0 g protein, 1 g carbohydrates, 2 g fat, 0 mg cholesterol, 0 g fiber, 12 mg sodium

ENDIVE AND AVOCADO SALAD
WITH LEMON DRESSING

Avocados are in season in California and Florida during the winter months, and though the food miles may be a bit longer, their outstanding nutrition (a slew of phytochemicals for heart health and vitamin E for healthy skin, to name a few) and heart-healthy fats make them a wise trade—especially as part of your new delicious flexitarian lifestyle. Their heavy exterior means they don't need to be heavily packaged.

This recipe is inspired by a salad that I love from Ina Garten's *Barefoot Contessa* series. The refreshing contrast between smooth and creamy avocado, sharp endive, and tangy mustard is oh so satisfying.

> 1 tablespoon olive oil
>
> 1 tablespoon fresh lemon juice
>
> 1 teaspoon Dijon mustard
>
> 4 endives, rinsed and chopped
>
> ½ avocado, chopped
>
> Pinch of salt and freshly cracked pepper

In a medium bowl, whisk together the olive oil, lemon juice, and mustard. Add the endives and avocado and toss gently to coat. Season to taste with salt and pepper.

MAKES 2 SERVINGS

Per serving: 232 calories, 8 g protein, 23 g carbohydrates, 15 g fat, 0 mg cholesterol, 26 g fiber, 177 mg sodium

---

ORANGE AND AVOCADO SLICES

Toss 3 thin avocado slices with about ½ cup orange sections (about half of an orange).

MAKES 1 SERVING

Per serving: 76 calories, 1 g protein, 10 g carbohydrates, 4 g fat, 0 mg cholesterol, 5 g fiber, 2 mg sodium

EGGLESS EGG SALAD

Look no more for a fantastic "egg salad" recipe that uses tofu instead of eggs. This is easy and tasty, and can be a staple in grab-and-go lunches. This recipe is compliments of Fairweather Natural Foods in Park City, Utah. I am grateful that they shared it with me, as I've been a devotee ever since I first found it! The nutritional yeast adds flavor but also provides a rich source of protein and vitamin B_{12}, so it's best not to omit it. Enjoy in a whole wheat pita with ½ cup chopped or shredded seasonal vegetables.

¼ cup canola mayonnaise or vegan mayonnaise

1 teaspoon granulated garlic

1 tablespoon fresh chopped parsley

1 tablespoon nutritional yeast

1 teaspoon turmeric

¼ cup diced celery

½ teaspoon dried dill (or 1 teaspoon fresh if in season)

1 block extra-firm tofu, drained and chopped

Salt and freshly cracked pepper

In a medium bowl, mix together the mayonnaise, garlic, parsley, yeast, turmeric, celery, and dill until well combined. Add the tofu and gently fold into the mixture. Taste and season with salt and pepper.

MAKES 4 SERVINGS (⅔ CUP EACH)

Per serving: 214 calories, 10 g protein, 5 g carbohydrates, 17 g fat, 5 mg cholesterol, 2 g fiber, 112 mg sodium

---

WINTER ENDIVE SALAD
WITH ROASTED ROSEMARY CHICKEN

Top unlimited endive leaves with 3 ounces extra Roasted Rosemary Chicken (page 286), 1 tablespoon cashews, 1 tablespoon sunflower seeds, 2 tablespoons dried cherries, ½ cup rinsed and drained beans (kidney, navy, or chickpeas), 2 tablespoons chopped red onion, and ⅓ cup tangerine slices. Drizzle with 1 tablespoon Pomegranate Vinaigrette (page 278). Serve with 6 whole grain crackers.

MAKES 1 SERVING

Per serving: 449 calories, 30 g protein, 54 g carbohydrates, 14 g fat, 48 mg cholesterol, 15 g fiber, 105 mg sodium

PAN-SEARED BRUSSELS SPROUTS WITH GRUYÈRE

This super-easy and delicious preparation will go over well for even the most die-hard skeptics, and the cheese is used here to make it tasty and comforting. It's inspired by a recipe I love by chef Heidi Swanson. Look for small Brussels sprouts that are tightly closed; the larger ones don't cook as quickly and can be tougher. Because they taste best as soon as they're cooked, and it's so fast and foolproof, this is one recipe that you should make fresh each time.

24 small Brussels sprouts (about 2 pounds), washed, stems trimmed, and sliced in half

3 tablespoon olive oil

½ teaspoon salt

Freshly ground black pepper

¼ cup grated Gruyère, Parmesan, or local nutty-flavored cheese

2 tablespoons chopped pistachios or almonds

1. Place the Brussels sprouts in a medium bowl and toss with 2 tablespoons of the olive oil until coated.

2. Heat the remaining 1 tablespoon olive oil in a large skillet over medium heat. Place the Brussels sprouts in the pan flat side down (keep to a single layer), sprinkle with the salt and pepper, cover, and cook until just tender and the bottoms just begin to brown, about 5 minutes; *do not overcook*. You can taste one of the sprouts to gauge tenderness if need be. If still hard, cover and cook for a few more minutes.

3. Once just tender, uncover, increase the heat to medium-high, and cook until the flat sides are brown and caramelized, about 3 to 4 more minutes. Toss them once or twice to get nice browning on the rounded sides, too. Sprinkle with the cheese and nuts. Serve hot.

MAKES 5 SERVINGS (½ CUP EACH)

Per serving: 151 calories, 4 g protein, 8 g carbohydrates, 12 g fat, 6 mg cholesterol, 4 g fiber, 273 mg sodium

PUREED SWEET POTATOES WITH LIME

2 sweet potatoes, scrubbed and pricked with a fork
in several places

Juice of 1 lime

Pinch of salt and pepper

Preheat the oven to 375°F. Bake the sweet potatoes until soft, about 45 minutes. Remove and let cool. Scoop the flesh into a medium bowl and add the lime juice; mash well. Alternately, you can puree in a food processor for a whipped, smooth consistency. Add the salt and pepper and serve hot.

MAKES 2 SERVINGS

Per serving: 115 calories, 2 g protein, 27 g carbohydrates, 0 g fat, 0 mg cholesterol, 5 g fiber, 280 mg sodium

---

HEALTHY TRAIL MIX

1 cup raw almonds

1 cup dried cranberries, raisins, or cherries
(unsweetened)

½ cup pumpkin or sunflower seeds

¼ cup 70% cacao chocolate chips

2 cups whole-grain Os cereal

Place all ingredients in an airtight, reusable container and mix well. Put individual servings in reusable 1 ounce containers.

MAKES 15 SERVINGS (⅛ CUP)

Per serving: 143 calories, 13 g carbohydrates, 3 g fiber, 4 g protein, 1 mg cholesterol, 8 g fat, 30 mg sodium

WARM PINK LENTILS

Lentils are a fantastic addition to your eating style because they are loaded with fiber, rich in folate, and high in protein. Even more important, they help regulate blood sugar (by slowing the rate at which glucose is absorbed) and are incredibly versatile in cooking. There are many types of lentils, so feel free to serve whichever kind you like best. Personally, I like the red and the French lentils (which are smaller, greenish lentils) because of their creamy texture, beautiful color, and quicker cooking time.

> 1½ cups pink lentils, rinsed
>
> 4 cups broth or water (can add a pinch of salt if using water)
>
> ½ onion, chopped

In a medium saucepan, place the lentils, broth, and onion. Simmer until tender, about 30 minutes. Add more liquid if necessary. Taste and adjust the seasoning.

MAKES 9 SERVINGS (⅔ CUP EACH)

Per serving: 124 calories, 8 g protein, 21 g carbohydrates, 1 g fat, 0 mg cholesterol, 4 g fiber, 203 mg sodium

---

PORK TENDERLOIN WITH POMEGRANATE VINAIGRETTE

Enjoy 4 ounces of grilled, baked, or broiled organic local pork tenderloin drizzled with 2 tablespoons Pomegranate Vinaigrette (page 278). Serve with 1 cup of roasted cauliflower and 1 cup Warm Pink Lentils (above).

MAKES 1 SERVING

Per serving: 226 calories, 30 g protein, 3 g carbohydrates, 10 g fat, 83 mg cholesterol, 0 g fiber, 101 mg sodium

WHOLE WHEAT PENNE WITH ROASTED CAULIFLOWER AND KALE ALMOND PESTO

Here's another recipe that comes compliments of my friend Chef Keith Snow from Harvest Eating. This dish highlights all that is so delicious and hearty about lean and green eating in wintertime. Roast the cauliflower and shallots in advance (using the basic method from the Roasted Fall Vegetables, page 286), and the dish is a cinch.

KALE ALMOND PESTO

2 cups steamed, chopped kale (remove tough stems prior to steaming)

½ cup almonds, toasted

2 tablespoons minced shallots

1 clove garlic, minced

Kosher salt

4 tablespoons Parmigiano-Reggiano cheese

Black pepper

½ cup extra virgin olive oil

PASTA

5 tablespoons extra virgin olive oil

1 cup roasted cauliflower

½ cup roasted shallots

½ pound whole wheat penne pasta (cooked)

2 tablespoons minced fresh chives (optional)

1 teaspoon orange zest

1 tablespoon orange juice

Salt and freshly cracked pepper

3 tablespoons grated Parmesan cheese (optional)

1. *To make the pesto:* In the bowl of a food processor, add the kale, almonds, shallots, garlic, salt to taste, cheese, and pepper to taste.

2. Pulse several times to combine, then drizzle in the olive oil.

3. Taste and adjust the seasoning.

4. Refrigerate for up to 1 week. Freeze remaining pesto in ice-cube trays for future use.

5. *To make the pasta:* In a large skillet over medium heat, place 3 tablespoons of the olive oil, the cauliflower, and the shallots. Cook, stirring frequently, for 2 minutes, then add the cooked pasta. Stir to combine.

6. Add 3 tablespoons of the pesto and stir often to prevent sticking. Add 1 tablespoon chives, if desired, and the orange zest and continue stirring. Add the orange juice and salt and pepper to taste. Ladle into bowls, top with the remaining 1 tablespoon of chives, if desired, and serve. (If you have any remaining cheese left in your Prescription, add 1 tablespoon Parmesan per serving.)

MAKES 3 SERVINGS (PLUS 3 CUPS PESTO)

Per serving: 450 calories, 12 g protein, 31 g carbohydrates, 34 g fat, 12 mg cholesterol, 7 g fiber, 467 mg sodium

---

STEAMED FISH WITH KALE ALMOND PESTO

When my grill is covered with 4 feet of snow (which is about 4 months of the year), steamed fish is comforting and warm in winter, easy to make, and a low-fat preparation. This dish is another delicious way to enjoy any remaining Kale Almond Pesto!

> **4 ounces green fish**
>
> **1 teaspoon olive oil**
>
> **Salt and freshly cracked pepper**
>
> **1 onion slice**
>
> **1 lemon slice**
>
> **2 tablespoons Kale Almond Pesto**

1. Preheat the oven to 375°F.

2. Place a large square of parchment paper on a baking sheet or in a casserole dish. Place the fish on the parchment paper. Drizzle the olive oil over the fish and add a pinch of salt and pepper. Top with the onion and lemon. Fold up the parchment paper so the fish is sealed into this "pouch."

3. Bake until steamed and cooked through, about 15 minutes. Use caution when opening the pouch, as it may be hot.

4. Top with the pesto and serve.

MAKES 1 SERVING

Per serving: 279 calories, 33 g protein, 6 g carbohydrates, 13 g fat, 56 mg cholesterol, 2 g fiber, 151 mg sodium

SEARED WILD SALMON WITH SUMMER PESTO

Enjoy 4 ounces of grilled or baked wild Alaskan salmon (ideally, frozen at sea) topped with 1 tablespoon of your thawed frozen summer pesto. (If you don't have pesto, you can drizzle with 1 tablespoon Pomegranate Vinaigrette [page 278] for a delicious alternative.)

MAKES 1 SERVING

Per serving: 251 calories, 28 g protein, 1 g carbohydrates, 15 g fat, 78 mg cholesterol, 0 g fiber, 187 mg sodium

---

ROASTED ROSEMARY CHICKEN WITH ROASTED FALL VEGETABLES

This, too, was inspired by an Ina Garten dish. To me, nothing is more comforting than a roast chicken dinner after a long day when it's cold out. You can use any combo of your favorite seasonal vegetables here. Make sure all the veggies are cut into roughly the same size, so they all will be ready at the same time.

CHICKEN

1 organic local roasting chicken (5–6 pounds)

1 lemon, halved

1 head garlic, halved

3–4 branches rosemary (thyme and parsley also work well)

2 tablespoons olive oil

1 yellow onion, quartered

Salt and freshly cracked pepper

ROASTED FALL VEGETABLES

1 organic local roasting
1 butternut squash (about 2 pounds), peeled and cubed

2 parsnips, peeled and cubed

1 large carrot, peeled and cubed

¼ cup olive oil

1 teaspoon salt

Freshly ground pepper

1. *To make the chicken:* Preheat the oven to 400°F. Rinse and pat dry the chicken, then place in a roasting pan. Stuff the lemon, garlic, and rosemary into the cavity of the chicken and either fold the legs closed (I am often too

lazy to do the official "tie with twine") or tie with kitchen string. Drizzle the chicken with the olive oil, rubbing it evenly over the outside of the chicken. Tuck the onion around the sides of the chicken. Season with salt and pepper. Roast for 1 to 1½ hours, or until a thermometer inserted into a breast registers 170°F and the juices run clear. Remove and let rest for about 10 minutes before slicing.

2. *To make the vegetables:* Place all ingredients on a baking sheet or in a casserole dish and toss together. When the chicken has about 30 minutes left to cook, place the vegetables in the oven. Roast alongside the chicken until the vegetables are tender, about 35 to 40 minutes.

MAKES 8 SERVINGS

Per 4-ounce serving (chicken only): 243 calories, 18 g protein, 1 g carbohydrates, 16 g fat, 78 mg cholesterol, 0 g fiber, 73 mg sodium

Per serving (vegetables only): 143 calories, 2 g protein, 21 g carbohydrates, 7 g fat, 0 mg cholesterol, 4 g fiber, 39 mg sodium

---

CINNAMON APPLE COMPOTE

Apples or pears work well in this delicious topping. You can make this in the fall, too, and use a splash of fresh local apple cider instead of the pear nectar.

> ¼ cup pear nectar
>
> 2 local apples (preferably sweet, not tart), peeled, cored, and diced
>
> ¼ teaspoon cinnamon
>
> Pinch of nutmeg

In a small saucepan, warm the nectar. Add the apples, cinnamon, and nutmeg and simmer until softened and slightly reduced, about 4 to 5 minutes. Serve warm or chilled.

MAKES 8 SERVINGS, ABOUT 2 CUPS (¼ CUP EACH)

Per serving: 29 calories, 0 g protein, 8 g carbohydrates, 0 g fat, 0 mg cholesterol, 2 g fiber, 1 mg sodium

END NOTES

INTRODUCTION

1. G. Eshel and P. A. Martin, "Diet, Energy and Global Warming," *Earth Interactions* (2006) 10(9):1–17.

2. D. Pimentel and M. Pimentel, eds., *Food, Energy and Society* (Niwot, CO: University Press of Colorado, 1996).

CHAPTER 1

1. D. Pimentel et al., "Reducing Energy Inputs in the US Food System," *Human Ecology* (2008) DOI 10.1007/s10745-008-9184-3.

CHAPTER 2

1. Gary McWilliams, "U.S. Consumers Trade Down as Economic Angst Grows," *The Wall Street Journal,* July 11, 2008.

2. From Deborah Madison's foreword written for Carlo Petrini's *Slow Food: Collected Thoughts on Taste, Tradition, and the Honest Pleasures of Food* (White River Junction, VT: Chelsea Green Publishing Company, 2001).

3. Waste Resource Action Programme (WRAP). "The Food We Waste: A Study of the Amount, Types and Nature of the Food We Throw Away in UK Households." April 2008.

4. S. Brodjt, E. Chernoh, and G. Feenstra, *Assessment of Energy Use and Greenhouse Gas Emissions in the Food System: A Literature Review* (Davis, CA: Agricultural Sustainability Institute, University of California, Davis, 2007).

CHAPTER 3

1. "Carbon Footprint of Best Conserving Americans Is Still Double Global Average," *Science Daily,* April 29, 2008, http://www.sciencedaily.com/releases/2008/04/080428120658.htm. Accessed August 3, 2008.

2. David Pimentel, *Human Ecology* (2008) DOI: 10.1007/s10745-008-9184-3.

3. 2005 US Dietary Guidelines for Americans, Chapter 6, Fats, Table 10.

4. David Pimentel and Marcia Pimentel, "The Future of American Agriculture," in *Sustainable Food Systems,* ed. Dietrich Knorr (Westport, CT: AVI Publishing Co., 1983).

5. K. J. Kramer, et al. "Greenhouse Gas Emissions Related to Dutch Food Consumption." *Energy Policy* (1999) 27: 203-16; and C. L. Weber and H. S. Matthews, "Food Miles and the Relative Cclimate Impacts of Food Choices in the United States." *Environ Sci Technol* (2008) 42(10): 3508–13.

6. USDA's Economic Research Service.

7. Elizabeth Rogers and Thomas Kostigen, *The Green Book* (New York: Three Rivers Press, 2007), 70.

8. Bon Appetit Management Company Low Carbon Diet Initiative, www.eatlowcarbon.org, accessed June 30, 2008, and The Food Processor, ESHA version 8.8, December 2006, accessed July 8, 2008. USDA CALCULATOR: http://www.nal.usda.gov/fnic/foodcomp/search/index.html.

9. USDA Economic Research Service.

10. Brian Wansink, "Environmental Factors That Increase the Food Intake and Consumption Volume of Unknowing Consumers," *Annual Review of Nutrition* (July 2004) 24: 455–79, and J. A. Ello-Martin et al., "Increasing the Portion Size of a Unit Food Increases Energy Intake," *Appetite* (2002) 39:74.

11. Maura L. Scott, Stephen M. Nowlis, et al. "The Effects of Reduced Food Size and Package Size on the Consumption Behavior of Restrained and Unrestrained Eaters." *J Cons Res* (2008) 35(3).

12. J. F. Hollis et al., "Weight Loss during the Intensive Intervention Phase of the Weight-Loss Maintenance Trial," *Am J Prev Med* (2008) 35(2):118–26.

13. J. S. Dukes, "Burning Buried Sunshine: Human Consumption of Ancient Solar Energy," *Climatic Change* (2003) 61(1–2):31–44

14. USDA Economic Research Service.

15. George A. Bray, Samara Joy Nielsen, and Barry M. Popkin, "Consumption of High-Fructose Corn Syrup in Beverages May Play a Role in the Epidemic of Obesity," *Am J Clin Nutr* (2004) 79(4):537–43.

16. M. B. Schulze et al., "Sugar-Sweetened Beverages, Weight Gain, and Incidence of Type 2 Diabetes in Young and Middle-Aged Women," *JAMA* (2004) 292:927–34.

17. S. P. Fowler, 65th Annual Scientific Sessions, American Diabetes Association, San Diego, June 10–14, 2005; Abstract 1058-P, Sharon P. Fowler, MPH, University of Texas Health Science Center School of Medicine, San Antonio; T.L. Davidson, "Artificial Sweeteners May Damage Diet Efforts," *Int. J. Obes* (July 2004) 28:933–55.

18. "Carbon Footprint." A report in December 2007 by Tate & Lyle Company. http://www.sucrose.com/bsst/2008agm1.pdf. Accessed August 2, 2008.

19. David Pimentel and Marcia Pimental, *Food, Energy, and Society* (New York: John Wiley and Sons, 1979).

20. Michael Pollan, *The Omnivore's Dilemma* (New York: Penguin Press, 2006), 115.

21. Michael Oshman interview with WBUR's Meghna Chakrabarti, 12, 2007. "And how would you like that cooked? . . . Green." http://www.wbur.org/news/local/dininggreen/story.asp.

22. CSFII 1994, and CSFII 1995.

23. For an in-depth look at the food psychology of eating, see Brian Wansink, *Mindless Eating: Why We Eat More Than We Think* (New York: Bantam Books, 2006).

24. Isaac Wolf, "Restaurant Menu Promises Buried in Calories, Fat." SeattlePi. com, May 22, 2008. Accessed on November 10, 2008. http://seattlepi.nwsource.com/local/364097_calories22.html

25. Bruce Horovitz, "Can Restaurants Go Green, Earn Green?" *USA Today* online. Posted 5/19/2008. http://www.usatoday.com/money/industries/environment/2008-05-15-green-restaurants-eco-friendly_N.htm. Accessed August 3, 2008.

26. Elizabeth Rogers and Thomas Kostigen, *The Green Book* (New York: Three Rivers Press, 2007), 57.

CHAPTER 4

1. G. Turner-McGrievy et al., "A Two-Year Randomized Weight Loss Trial Comparing a Vegan Diet to a More Moderate Low-Fat Diet," *Obesity* (2007) 15:2276–81.

2. F. M. Sacks et al., "Effects of Ingestion of Meat on Plasma Cholesterol of Vegetarians," *JAMA* (1981) 246:640–44; A. Ascherio et al., "Prospective Study Nutrition Factors, Blood Pressure and Hypertension among US Women," *Hypertension* (1996) 27:1065–72; A. Chao et al., "Meat Consumption and Risk of Colorectal Cancer," *JAMA* (2005) 293:172–82; T. Key and G. Davey, "Prevalence of Obesity Is Lower in People Who Do Not Eat Meat," *BMJ* (1996) 313:816–17.

3. CSPI Nutrition Action Newsletter, "New Year's Resolutions," January/February (2007) 32(1):3–6.

4. Worldwatch Institute Web site. http://www.worldwatch.org/node/791. Accessed August 4, 2008.

5. USDA Calculator: http://www.nal.usda.gov/fnic/foodcomp/search/index.html. Prices taken from Super Stop & Shop Supermarket, 37 Enon Street, Beverly, MA 01915, June 9, 2008, and Bob's Red Mill Website: http://www.bobsredmill.com/catalog/index.php?action=express. Accessed June 9, 2008.

6. American Heart Association.

7. See the research outlined in Walter Willett, MD, and the Harvard School of Public Health, *Eat, Drink, and Be Healthy* (New York: Simon and Schuster, 2001), and Bradley J. Wilcox, Craig Wilcox, and Makoto Suzuki, *The Okinawa Program* (New York: Three Rivers Press, 2001).

8. T. Colin Campbell and Thomas M. Campbell II, *The China Study: Startling Implications for Diet, Weight Loss, and Long-Term Health* (Dallas, TX: BenBella Books, 2004).

9. "Rearing Cattle Produces More Greenhouse Gases Than Driving Cars, UN Report Warns," UN News Centre, November 29, 2006.

10. http://www.greenprogress.com/carbon_footprint_calculator.php.

11. Eshel and Martin, 2006.

12. Results of a 2003 Vegetarian Resource Group Harris Interactive poll, http://www.vrg.org/journal/vj2003issue3/vj2003issue3poll.htm.

13. A. Carlsson-Kanyma et al., *Energy Use in the Food Sector* (Stockholm, Sweden: Stockholm University, 2000).

14. O. Akifumi et al., "Evaluating Environmental Impacts of the Japanese Beef Cow-Calf System by the Life Cycle Assessment Method," *Animal Science Journal* (2007) 78(4):424–32.

15. M. Jacobson, *Six Arguments for a Greener Diet,* (Center for Science in the Public Interest, 2006).

16. Eshel and Martin, 2006.

17. M. Nestle, *What to Eat,* p. 139.

18. M. Jacobson, *Six Arguments for a Greener Diet.*

19. I. Hoffman, "Ecological Impact of a High-Meat, Low-Meat and Ovo-Lacto Vegetarian Diet," presentation, Fourth International Congress on Vegetarian Nutrition, April 8–11, 2002, Loma Linda University, School of Public Health.

20. US Dept. of Energy, 2004b. "Emissions of Greenhouse Gases in the United States 2003," Report No. DEO/EIA-0573(2003), December 13, 2004.

21. M. Jacobson, *Six Arguments,* p. 83.

22. http://www.cspinet.org/EatingGreen/calculator.html

23. Mayer and Rawitscher, 1979.

CHAPTER 5

1. T. T. Fung et al., "Dietary Patterns and the Risk of Coronary Heart Disease in Women," *Arch Intern Med* (2001), 161:1857–62; F. B. Hu et al., "Prospective Study of Major Dietary Patterns and Risk of Coronary Heart Disease in Men," *Am J Clin Nutr* (2000) 72:912–21.

2. G. Eshel and P.A. Martin, "Diet, Energy, and Global Warming," *Earth Interactions* (2006) 10(9):1–17.

3. Eshel and Martin, 2006.

4. Ute Nothlings, "Heavy Consumption of Processed Meats Linked to Increased Risk for Pancreatic Cancer," Cancer Research Center, University of Hawaii, Honolulu. Presented April 20, 2005, at the 96th Annual Meeting of the American Association for Cancer Research.

5. S. C. Larsson and A. Wolk, "Meat Consumption and Risk of Colorectal Cancer: A Meta-Analysis of Prospective Studies," *Int J Cancer* (2006) 119(11):2657–64; S. C. Larsson et al., "Processed Meat Consumption and Stomach Cancer Risk: A Meta-Analysis," *Int J Cancer* (2006) 98(15):1078–87.

6. Eshel and Martin, 2006.

7. Michael Shuman, "On the Lamb: Local vs. Global Food's Environmental Impact," http://www.bioneers.org/node/2178.

8. D. K. Asami et al., "Comparison of the Total Phenolic and Ascorbic Acid Content of Freeze-Dried and Air-Dried Marionberry, Strawberry, and Corn Grown Using Conventional, Organic, and Sustainable Agricultural Practices," *J Ag Food Chem* (2003) 51(5):1237–41.

9. D. M. Barrett et al., "Qualitative and Nutritional Differences in Processing Tomatoes Grown under Commercial Organic and Conventional Production Systems," *Journal of Food Science* (2007) 72(9):C441–51.

10. Heller and Keoleian, 2000.

11. N. El-Hage Scialabba and C. Hattam, eds., *Organic Agriculture, Environment, and Food Security* (Rome: UN Food and Agriculture Organization, 2002).

12. The Fertilizer Institute, http://www.tfi.org.

13. D. Pimentel et al., "Environmental, Energetic, and Economic Comparisons of Organic and Conventional Farming Systems," *Bioscience* (July 2005) 55(7):573–82.

14. David Pimentel, "Impacts of Organic Farming on the Efficiency of Energy Use in Agriculture: An Organic Center State of Science Review" (Ithaca, NY: Cornell University, The Organic Center, 2006).

15. Ibid.

16. *Six Arguments for a Greener Diet,* CSPI, p. 83.

17. C. Cederberg and M. Stadig, "System Expansion and Allocation in Life Cycle Assessment of Milk and Beef Production," *International Journal of Life Cycle Assessment* (2003) 8(6):350–56.

18. J. Reganold et al., "Sustainability of Three Apple Production Systems," *Nature* (2001) 410:926–30; P. Mäder et al., "Soil Fertility and Biodiversity in Organic Farming," *Science* (2002) 296:1694–97.

19. Kelly Myers, "Grass Fed Lamb: Which Foods Are You Willing to Pay Top Dollar For?" May 6, 2008. http://www.culinate.com/columns/front_burner/grass_fed_lamb.

CHAPTER 6

1. F. Hu et al., "Fish and Omega-3 Fatty Acid Intake and Risk of Coronary Heart Disease in Women," *JAMA* (2002) 287:1815–21; C. M. Albert et al., "Blood Levels of Long-Chain n-3 Fatty Acids and the Risk of Sudden Death," *N Engl J Med* (2002) 346:1113–18.

2. USDA Calculator: http://www.nal.usda.gov/fnic/foodcomp/search/index.html. Accessed June 5, 2008.

3. The Worldwatch Institute, "2008 State of the World: Innovations for a Sustainable Economy."

4. Center for Science in the Public Interest, *Nutrition Action Healthletter,* David Schart, "Farmed Salmon under Fire," June 2004.

5. P. H. Tyedmers et al., "Fueling Global Fishing Fleets," *AMBIO: A Journal of the Human Environment* (2005) 34(8):635–38.

6. This figure was provided by chef Rick Moonen, owner of Seafood Las Vegas, and one of the leading chefs focusing on sustainable seafood choices, at a panel discussion at the Monterey Bay Aquarium Sustainable Seafood Symposium, May 2008, Monterey, CA.

7. R. Hites et al., "Global Assessment of Organic Contaminants in Farmed Salmon," *Science* (2004) 303:226–29; M. D. L. Easton et al., "Preliminary Examination of Contaminant Loadings in Farmed Salmon, Wild Salmon, and Commercial Salmon Feed," *Chemosphere* (2002) 46:1053–74.

8. Marion Burros, "Stores Say Wild Salmon, but Tests Say Farm Bred," *The New York Times,* April 10, 2005.

9. C. A. Daley, et al. "A literature review of the value-added nutrients found in grass-fed beef products." College of Agriculture, California State University; and D. C. Rule, et al., "Comparison of Muscle Fatty Acid Profiles and Cholesterol Concentrations of Bison, Beef Cattle, Elk and Chicken." *J Anim Sci* (2002) 80(5): 1202-11.

10. USDA nutrient database: http://www.nal.usda.gov/fnic/foodcomp/search/.

CHAPTER 7

1. S. Berkow and N. Barnard, "Vegetarian Diets and Weight Status," *Nutr Reviews* (2006) 64(4):175–88.

2. P. N. Appleby et al., "Hypertension and Blood Pressure among Meat Eaters, Fish Eaters, Vegetarians, and Vegans in EPIC-Oxford," *Public Health Nutr* (2002) 5:645–54.

3. David Pimentel and Marcia Pimentel, "Sustainability of Meat-Based and Plant-Based Diets and the Environment," *Am J Clin Nutr* (2003) 78(3):661S–62S.

4. *The Green Book,* p. 71.

5. J. Sabate, "Nut Consumption and Body Weight," *Am J Clin Nutr* (2003) 78(3):647S–50; K. McManus, L. Antinoro, F. Sacks, "A Randomised Controlled Trial of a Moderate-Fat, Low-Energy Diet with a Low-Fat, Low-Energy Diet for Weight Loss in Overweight Adults," *Int J Obes* 25(5):1503–11.

6. F. B. Hu et al., "Frequent Nut Consumption and Risk of Coronary Heart Disease in Women: Prospective Cohort Study," *BMJ* (1998) 317:1341–45; J. L. Ellsworth, "Frequent Nut Intake and Risk of Death from Coronary Heart Disease and All Causes in Postmenopausal Women: The Iowa Women's Health Study," *Nutr Metab Cardiovasc Dis* (2001) 11(6):372—7; and Jiang et al., "Nut and Peanut Butter Consumption and Risk of Type 2 Diabetes in Women," *JAMA* (2002) 288:2554–60.

7. D. Zambon et al., "Substituting Walnuts for Monounsaturated Fat Improves the Serum Lipid Profile of Hypercholesterolemic Men and Women," *Circulation* (2004) 109(13):1609–14.

8. http://www.nutnutrition.com/allaboutnuts/pistachio.htm.

9. R. E. Ostlund et al., "Effects of Trace Components of Dietary Fat on Cholesterol Metabolism: Phytosterols, Oxysterols, and Squalene," *Nutr Rev* (2002) 60(11):349–59.

CHAPTER 8

1. Willett, 2001.

2. A. Lanou and N. Barnard, "Dairy and Weight Loss Hypothesis: An evaluation of the Clinical Trials," *Nutrition Reviews* (May 2008) 66(5):272–79.

3. David Schardt, "Milking the Data: Does Dairy Burn More Fat? Don't Bet Your Bottom on It," *Nutrition Action Healthletter,* September 2005.

4. T.R. Dhiman, "Conjugated Linoleic Acid: A Food for Cancer Prevention." Proceedings from the 2000 Intermountain Nutrition Conference, pages 103–21.

5. USDA calculator: http://www.nal.usda.gov/fnic/foodcomp/search/index.html; The Food Processor, ESHA version 8.8, December 2006, accessed June 5, 2008.

6. E. Thom et al., "Conjugated Linoleic Acid Reduces Body Fat in Healthy Exercising Humans," *J Intl Med Res* (2001) 29(5):392–96; H. Blankson et al., "Conjugated Linoleic Acid Reduces Body Fat Mass in Overweight and Obese Humans," *J Nutr* (2000) 130(12):2943–48; U. Risérus et al., "Supplementation with Conjugated Linoleic Acid Causes Isomer-Dependent Oxidative Stress and Elevated C-Reactive Protein: A Potential Link to Fatty Acid-Induced Insulin Resistance," *Circulation* (2002) 106(15):1925–29; U. Risérus U et al., "Treatment with Dietary Trans10cis12 Conjugated Linoleic Acid Causes Isomer-Specific Insulin Resistance in Obese Men with the Metabolic Syndrome," *Diabetes Care* (2002) 25(9):1516–21.

7. A. Aro et al., Kuopio University, Finland; P. Bougnoux; F. Lavillonniere; and E. Riboli, "Inverse Relation between CLA in Adipose Breast Tissue and Risk of Breast Cancer. A Case-Control Study in France," *Inform* (1999) 10(5):S43.

8. L. Rist et al., "Influence of Organic Diet on the Amount of Conjugated Linoleic Acids in Breast Milk," *British J of Nutr* (June 2007) 97: 735–43.

9. L. Lavillonniere et al., "Analysis of Conjugated Linoleic Acid Isomers and Content in French Cheeses," *J Am Oil Chem Soc* (1998) 75(3):343–52.

10. R. J. Dewhurst, et al., "Comparison of Grass and Legume Silages for Milk Production. Production Responses with Different Levels of Concentrate." *J Dairy Sci* (2003) 86:2598–611.

11. S.K. Jensen, "Quantitative Secretion and Maximal Secretion Capacity of Retinol, Beta-Carotene and Alpha-Tocopherol into Cows' Milk," *J Dairy Res* (1999) 66(4):511–22; J. Robertson and C. Fanning, "Omega-3 Polyunsaturated Fatty Acids in Organic and Conventional Milk," 2004: University of Aberdeen, Institute of Grassland and Environmental Research, Aberystwyth, Wales; P. Bergamo et al., "Fat-Soluble Vitamin Contents and Fatty Acid Composition in Organic and Conventional Italian Dairy Products," *Food Chemistry* (2003) 82:625–31.

12. C. Van Niel et al., "Lactobacillus Therapy for Acute Infectious Diarrhea in Children: A Meta-Analysis," *Pediatrics* (2002) 109:678–84; H. Szymanski, J. Pejcz, M. Jawien et al., "Treatment of Acute Infectious Diarrhea in Infants and Children with a Mixture of Three *Lactobacillus rhamnosus* Strains—A Randomized, Double-Blind, Placebo-Controlled Trial," *Aliment Pharmacol Ther* (2006) 23:247–53; K.

Kajander, E. Myllyluoma, M. Rajilić-Stojanović, et al., "Clinical Trial: Multispecies Probiotic Supplementation Alleviates the Symptoms of Irritable Bowel Syndrome and Stabilizes Intestinal Microbiota," *Aliment Pharmacol Ther* (2008) 27:48–57.

13. M.E. Falagas et al., "Probiotics for Prevention of Recurrent Vulvovaginal Candidiasis: A Review," *J Antimicrob Chemother* (2006) 58:266–72.

14. Eshel and Martin, 2005.

15. US Dept. of Energy, Energy Information Administration, 2004b: "Emissions of Greenhouse Gases in the United States 2003," Report No. DOE/EIA-0573(2003), December 13, 2004.

16. Rogers and Kostigen, 67.

17. A. Renehan et al., "Insulin-Like Growth Factor (IGF-1), IGF Binding Protein-3, and Cancer Risk: Systematic Review and Meta-Regression Analysis," *Lancet* (2004) 363:1346–53.

18. "Energy Use in Organic Farming Systems ADAS Consulting for MAFF," Project OF0182, DEFRA, London, 2001.

19. A.J. Wenzel et al., "A 12-Week Egg Intervention Increases Serum Zeaxanthin and Macular Pigment Optical Density in Women," *J Nutr* (2006) 136:2568–73.

20. Willet, p. 64.

CHAPTER 9

1. M. Purba et al., "Skin Wrinkling; Can Food Make a Difference?" *J Am Coll Nutr* (2001) 20(1):71–80.

2. B. Dawson-Hughes et al., "Alkaline Diets Favor Lean Tissue Mass in Older Adults," *Am J Clin Nutr* (2008) 87(3):662–65.

3. James A. Joseph, Daniel A. Nadeau, and Anne Underwood, *The Color Code: A Revolutionary Eating Plan for Optimum Health* (New York: Hyperion, 2002).

4. David Pimentel and Marcia Pimentel, "The Future of American Agriculture," in *Sustainable Food Systems,* ed. Dietrich Knorr (Westport, CT: AVI Publishing Co., 1983).

5. C. Weber and H. Matthews, "Food Miles and the Relative Climate Impacts of Food Choices in the United States," *Environ Sci Technol.* Web release date April 16, 2008.

6. Field to Plate Web site: http://www.fieldtoplate.com/guide.php. Accessed June 9, 2008.

7. Pirog et al., "Checking the Food Odometer: Comparing Food Miles for Local versus Conventional Produce Sales to Iowa Institutions," Leopold Center for Sustainable Agriculture, Iowa State University, July 2003.

8. Ibid.

9. Weber and Matthews, "Food Miles," April 16, 2008.

10. Ibid.

11. James McWilliams, "Moveable Feast: Eating Local Isn't Always the Greenest Option," *Texas Observer*, August 10, 2007. http://www.texasobserver.org/article.php?aid=25646.

12. M.M. Blank and B. Burdick, "Food (Miles) for Thought: Energy Balance for Locally Grown versus Imported Apple Fruit," *Environmental Science and Pollution Research* (2005) 12(3):125–27.

13. Elizabeth Rosenthal, "Environmental Cost of Shipping Groceries around the World," *The New York Times,* April 26, 2008.

14. Diane Welland, "5 New Exotic Fruits: How Super Good for You Are They?" *Environmental Nutrition* (June 2008) 31(6):2.

15. The Food Processor, ESHA version 8.8, December 2006. Accessed June 13, 2008.

16. S Brodt, E. Chernoh, and G. Feenstra, "Assessment of Energy Use and Greenhouse Gas Emissions in the Food System: A Literature Review," Agricultural Sustainability Institute, University of California Davis, November 2007.

CHAPTER 10

1. P. Cotton et al., "Dietary Sources of Nutrients among US Adults, 1994 to 1996," *J Am Diet Assoc* (2004) 104(6):921–30.

2. H. Katcher et al., "The Effects of a Whole Grain–Enriched Hypocaloric Diet on Cardiovascular Disease Risk Factors in Men and Women with Metabolic Syndrome," *Am J Clin Nutr* (2008) 87(1):79–90.

3. David Pimentel and Marcia Pimentel, *Food, Energy and Society* (New York: John Wiley and Sons, 1979).

CHAPTER 11

1. P. Garcia-Lorda et al., "Nut Consumption, Body Weight and Insulin Resistance," *Eur J Clin Nutr* (2003) 57, Suppl. 1, S8–S11; K. McManus, L. Antinoro, and F. Sacks, "A Randomized Controlled Trial of a Moderate Fat, Low-Energy Diet with a Low-Fat, Low-Energy Diet for Weight Loss in Overweight Adults," *Int J Obes* (2001) 25(5):1503–11; L.S. Piers et al., "Substitution of Saturated with Monounsaturated Fat in a 4-Week Diet Affects Body Weight and Composition of Overweight and Obese Men," *British J Nutr* (2003) 90:717–27; R. Jiang et al., "Nut and Peanut Butter Consumption and Risk of Type 2 Diabetes in Women," *JAMA* (2002) 288:2554–60.

2. Several studies have found that diets rich in heart-healthy fats can help with weight loss. K. McManus, L. Antinoro, and F. Sacks, "A Randomized Controlled Trial of a Moderate Fat, Low-Energy Diet with a Low-Fat, Low-Energy Diet for Weight Loss in Overweight Adults," *Int J Obes* (2001) 25(5):1503–11; L. S. Piers et al., "Substitution of Saturated with Monounsaturated Fat in a 4-Week Diet Affects Body Weight and Composition of Overweight and Obese Men," *British J Nutr* (2003) 90:717–27.

3. Wake Forest University Baptist Medical Center, "Trans Fat Leads to Weight Gain Even on Same Total Calories, Animal Study Shows," *ScienceDaily,* June 19,

2006 (accessed) June 9, 2008 http://www.sciencedaily.com/releases/2006/06/060619 133024.htm.

4. H. Kaunitz and C.S. Dayrit, "Coconut Oil Consumption and Coronary Heart Disease," *Philippine J Int Med* (1992) 30:165–71; G.L. Blackburn et al., "A Reevaluation of Coconut Oil's Effect on Serum Cholesterol and Atherogenesis," *J of the Philippine Med Assoc* (1989) 65:144–52; R.F. Florentino and A.R. Aquinaldo, "Diet and Cardiovascular Disease in the Philippines," *Philippine Journal of Coconut Studies* (1987) 12:56–70.

5. A. Dannenberg et al., "Economic and Environmental Costs of Obesity. The Impact on Airlines," *Am J Prev Med* (2004) 27(3):264.

6. S. Jacobson and L.A. McLay, "The Economic Impact of Obesity on Automobile Fuel Consumption," *Engineering Economist,* winter 2006. http://www.entrepreneur.com/ tradejournals/article/156363600_4.html. Accessed August 25, 2008.

CHAPTER 12

1. B. Burton-Freeman et al., "Plasma Cholecystokinin Is Associated with Subjective Measures of Satiety in Women," *Amer J Clin Nutr* (2002) 76:659–67.

2. C. Marmonier et al., "Snacks Consumed in a Non-Hungry State Have Poor Satiating Efficiency: Influence of Snack Composition on Substrate Utilization and Hunger," *Amer J Clin Nutr* (2002) 76:518–28.

3. Gidon Eshel and Pamela A. Martin, "Diet, Energy, and Global Warming," *Earth Interactions* (2006) 10:1–17.

4. A. Carlsson-Kanyama et al., "Food and Life Cycle Energy Inputs; Consequences of Diet and Ways to Increase Efficiency," *Ecological Economics* (2003) 44:293–307.

5. Brian Wansink, "Environmental Factors That Increase the Food Intake and Consumption Volume of Unknowing Consumers," *Annual Review of Nutrition* (July 2004) 24:455–79; J.A. Ello-Martin et al., "Increasing the Portion Size of a Unit Food Increases Energy Intake," *Appetite* (2002) 39:74.

6. V.E. Pudel and M. Oetting, "Eating in the Laboratory: Behavioral Aspects of the Positive Energy Balance," *Int J Obesity* (1977) 1:369–86.

7. B. Wansink and K. Junyong, "Bad Popcorn in Big Buckets: Portion Size Can Influence Intake as Much as Taste," *J Nutr Ed Beh* (2005) 37(5):242–45.

8. Gary Hirshberg, "Seven Cows and a Dream," *Newsweek,* February 25, 2008, E6.

CHAPTER 13

1. http://www.health.gov/dietaryguidelines/dga2005/report/.

2. D.P. DiMeglio and R.D. Mattes, "Liquid Versus Solid Carbohydrate: Effects on Food Intake and Body Weight," *International Journal of Obesity* (2000) 24: 794–800.

3. S.P. Fowler, 65th Annual Scientific Sessions, American Diabetes Association, San Diego, June 10–14, 2005; Abstract 1058-P, Sharon P. Fowler, MPH, University

of Texas Health Science Center School of Medicine, San Antonio; and T.L. Davidson, "Artificial Sweeteners May Damage Diet Efforts," *Int J Obes* (July 2004) 28:933–55.

4. Institute of Medicine, "Dietary Reference Intakes: Water, Potassium, Sodium, Chloride, and Sulfate," National Academies Press, February 11, 2004.

5. From *National Geographic*'s "The Human Footprint," aired April 13, 2008. http://ngcblog.nationalgeographic.com/ngcblog/2008/03/. Accessed August 28, 2008.

6. C. Fishman, "Message in a Bottle," *Fast Company,* Issue 117 (July 2007) 110.

7. Energy Information Administration: http://tonto.eia.doe.gov/oog/info/gdu/ gasdiesel.asp. Accessed June 17, 2008.

8. Janet Larson, "Bottled Water Boycotts: Back-to-the-Tap Movement Gains Momentum," December 7, 2007, Earth Policy Institute: http://www.earth-policy. org/Updates/2007/Update68.htm.

9. S.C. Renaud et al., "Alcohol and Mortality in Middle-Aged Men from Eastern France," *Epidemiology* (1998) 9(2):184–88.

10. T. Truelsen et al., "Intake of Beer, Wine, and Spirits and Risk of Stroke: The Copenhagen City Heart Study," *Stroke* (1998) 29(12):2467–72; Swedish Research Council, "Wine May Protect Against Dementia, Study Suggests" *ScienceDaily* (2008, April 13). Retrieved June 15, 2008, from http://www.sciencedaily.com.

11. T. Colman and P. Pastor, "Red, White and 'Green': The Cost of Carbon in the Global Wine Trade," American Association of Wine Economists, AAWE Working Paper No. 9. October 2007.

12. Ibid.

13. S.P. Fowler, 65th Annual Scientific Sessions, American Diabetes Association, Abstract 1058-P; T.L. Davidson, "Artificial Sweeteners," 933–55.

14. Pimentel, 1979.

15. http://www.recycle.novelis.com/Recycle/EN/Educators/Benefits+of+Alumi.

CHAPTER 14

1. Sid Kircheimer, "Coffee: The New Health Food?" Web MD feature. http://men. webmd.com/features/coffee-new-health-food. Accessed June 17, 2008.

2. A. Ascherio et al., "Coffee Consumption and Risk for Type 2 Diabetes Mellitus," *Annal Int Med* (2004) (1) 140:1–8; F. Bravi et al., "Coffee Drinking and Hepatocellular Carcinoma Risk: A Meta-Analysis," *Hepatology* (2007) 46(2):430–435; G.W. Ross et al., "Association of Coffee and Caffeine Intake with the Risk of Parkinson Disease," *JAMA* (2000) 283(20):2674–79.

3. P. Martin and J. Vinson, "Effects of Coffee Bean Aroma on the Rat Brain Stressed by Sleep Deprivation: A Selected Transcript and 2D Gel Based Proteome Analysis," *J Agric Food Chem* (2008) 56(12):4665–73.

4. International Food Information Council Web site: http://www.ific.org/. Accessed April 15, 2008.

5. USDA calculator: http://www.nal.usda.gov/fnic/foodcomp/search/index.html, accessed June 17, 2008; Starbucks Web site: http://www.starbucks.com/retail/nutrition_info.asp.

6. S.J. Duffy et al., "Short- and Long-Term Black Tea Consumption Reverses Endothelial Dysfunction in Patients with Coronary Artery Disease," *Circulation* (2001) 104:151-56; M. Isemura et al., "Tea Catechins and Related Polyphenols as Anti-Cancer Agents," *Biofactors* (2000) 13(1–4):81–85; J.M. Geleijnse et al., "Inverse Association of Tea and Flavonoid Intakes with Incident Myocardial Infarction: The Rotterdam Study," *Am J Clin Nutr* (May 2002) 75(5):880–86.

7. T. Nagao et al., "Ingestion of a Tea Rich in Catechins Leads to a Reduction in Body Fat and Malondialdehyde-Modified LDL in Men," *Am J Clin Nutr* (Jan 2005) 81(1):122–29; T. Nagao et al., "A Green Tea Extract High in Catechins Reduces Body Fat and Cardiovascular Risk in Humans," *Obesity* (Jun 2007) 15:1473–83.

8. C.H. Wu et al., "Epidemiological Evidence of Increased Bone Mineral Density in Habitual Tea Drinkers," *Arch Intern Med* (May 13, 2002) 162(9):1001–6.

9. K. Bruinsma, "Chocolate, Food or Drug?" *Journal of the American Dietetic Association* (1999) 99:1249–56.

10. V. Charalambos et al., "Effect of Dark Chocolate on Arterial Function in Healthy Individuals," *Am J Hypertens* (2005) 18:785–91; R. Allen et al., "Daily Consumption of a Dark Chocolate Containing Flavonols and Added Sterol Esters Affects Cardiovascular Risk Factors in a Normotensive Population with Elevated Cholesterol," *J Nutr* (2008) 138(4):725–31.

11. D. Taubert et al., "Effects of Low Habitual Cocoa Intake on Blood Pressure and Bioactive Nitric Oxide: A Randomized Controlled Trial," *JAMA* (2007) 298(1):49–60.

12. Rainforest Action Network Agribusiness campaign. http://ran.org/what_we_do/rainforest_agribusiness/about_the_campaign/. Accessed September 2, 2008.

13. O.H. Franco et al., "The Polymeal: A More Natural, Safer, and Probably Tastier (Than the Polypill) Strategy to Reduce Cardiovascular Disease by More Than 75%," *BMJ* (2004) 329:1447–50.

14. Pimentel, 1979.

15. *The Green Book,* p. 68.

16. Word Watch Institute. "The Price of Beef," *World Watch Magazine*, July/August 1994, Volume 7, No. 4.

17. Rainforest Action Network.

18. Greener Choices Web site, http://www.greenerchoices.org/products.cfm?product=coffee&pcat=food. Accessed April 20, 2008.

19. From the foreword (written by Deborah Madison) of *Slow Food: Collected Thoughts on Taste, Tradition and the Honest Pleasures of Food*, ed. Carlo Petrini, (White River Junction, VT: Chelsea Green Publishing Company, 2001).

INDEX

Underscored page references indicate sidebars and tables. **Boldface** references indicate illustrations.

A

Acorn squash
  Wild Rice Stuffed Acorn Squash, 267
ALA, 92
Alcohol, 39, 43–44, 47, 194–95. *See also* Beer; Wine
Almonds, 104
  Spinach Salad with Strawberries, Almonds, and Poppy Seeds, 242
  Steamed Fish with Kale Almond Pesto, 285
  Whole Wheat Penne with Roasted Cauliflower and Kale Almond Pesto, 284–85
Alpha-linoleic acid (ALA), 92
Animal products
  calculating impact of eating, 64
  health effects of, 59
  myth about, 66
  organic, 76–77
  reducing portions of, 54
Apples
  Cinnamon Apple Compote, 287
Appliances, energy-efficient, 26–27, 47
Apricots
  Apricot Stuffed with Goat Cheese, 248
Artificial sweeteners, 39, 43, 47, 180, 203
Asparagus
  Asparagus Salad with Sesame Ginger Vinaigrette, 240
  Grilled Asparagus with Lemon, 241
Avocados
  Endive and Avocado Salad with Lemon Dressing, 279
  Orange and Avocado Slices, 279

B

Bananas, "green," 219
Barley, 155
  Warm Barley and Quinoa Porridge with Soymilk, 236
Beans
  action plan for eating, 107
  Autumn Squash and Pinto Bean Chili with Cinnamon and Cumin, 263
  Farm Salad with Beans and Fingerling Potatoes, 254
  Fresh Corn, Pepper, and Black Bean Tacos, 257
  green benefits of, 102–3
  Hearty Winter Bean Chili, 277
  lean and green prescription for, 99
  lean benefits of, 100–102, 101
  serving suggestions for, 102
  Tabbouleh Salad with White Beans, 253
Beef
  calculating impact of eating, 64
  effects on rainforest, 218
  lean and green prescription for, 55
  organic grass-fed, 80
  reducing consumption of
    action plan for, 33–34
    green benefits of, 32–33, 33, 60–64
    lean benefits of, 30–32, 56–60
Beer, 187–88, 194–95
Beets
  Baby Beets with Orange Zest, 243
  Warmed Beets with Walnut Oil and Chopped Walnuts, 266
Belly fat, 148–49, 162–63
Berries. *See also specific berries*
  Chilled Oatmeal with Summer Fruit, 250
  Gorgeous Green Smoothie, 273
  Summer Smoothie, 250

Greenhouse gas emissions, effect of
food supply on, 4, 29
Greens
Fall Green Frittata, 261
Gorgeous Greens in a Flash, 265
"Greenwashing," 14, 178–79, 191

H

Health packs, for snacking, 170–71
Heart disease
death risk from, 86
eating style reducing, 59, 67, 215
High-fructose corn syrup (HFCS), 39,
43, 44, 45–46, 173, 180
Hummus, 102, 170
Cumin Lime Hummus, 254
Garlicky Edamame Hummus, 241
Hummus Wrap, 243

I

IGF-1, 120
Industrial food, 172–73, 173, 174, 175–76.
See also Convenience foods;
Processed foods
purging, from pantry, 22, 179–82
Inflammation, dietary fats and, 158,
159, 161–62, 162
Insulin-like growth factor 1 (IGF-1), 120

J

Juice, 198–99
grape, 194, 200
increasing green benefits of, 200–201
lean benefits of, 199
orange, 200, 219–20

K

Kale
Steamed Fish with Kale Almond
Pesto, 285
Whole Wheat Penne with Roasted
Cauliflower and Kale Almond
Pesto, 284–85

L

Labels, eco-chic food, 200, 219, 220
Lamb, 65, 72–74

L.E.A.N. Cheat Sheet, 154, 165, 178
Lean and Green Prescriptions, 11
Legumes, 98. See also Beans; Lentils
action plan for eating, 107
green benefits of, 102–3
lean and green prescription for, 99
lean benefits of, 100–102
Lemons
Endive and Avocado Salad with
Lemon Dressing, 279
Grilled Asparagus with Lemon, 241
Spring Lettuce Salad with Tuscan
Lemon Vinaigrette, 239
Tuscan Lemon Vinaigrette, 239
Lentils
Warm Pink Lentils, 283
Lettuce
Farm Salad with Beans and
Fingerling Potatoes, 254
Farm Salad with Hard-Boiled Egg,
254
Spring Lettuce Salad with Tuscan
Lemon Vinaigrette, 239
Limes
Cumin Lime Hummus, 254
Pureed Sweet Potatoes with Lime,
282
Localism
benefits of, 19, 22, 139–43
boundaries for, 143
for choosing
dairy products, 118–19, 166
produce, 131, 135–38
wine, 195
product space and, 156

M

Meats. See also specific meats
benefits of eating less, 100
red, 59, 60, 69–71
Mediterranean diet, 160
Menus, seasonal, 23
fall, 232–33
spring, 228–29
summer, 230–31
winter, 234–35
Milk
lean and green prescription for, 108
organic, 113, 114, 119, 120
weight-loss claims about, 112
Mini meals, weight loss and, 170